THE SENSES IN SELF, SOCIETY, AND CULTURE

The Senses in Self, Society, and Culture is the definitive guide to the sociological and anthropological study of the senses. Vannini, Waskul, and Gottschalk provide a comprehensive map of the social and cultural significance of the senses that is woven in a thorough analytical review of classical, recent, and emerging scholarship and grounded in original empirical data that deepens the review and analysis. By bridging cultural/qualitative sociology and cultural/humanistic anthropology, *The Senses in Self, Society, and Culture* explicitly blurs boundaries that are particularly weak in this field due to the ethnographic scope of much research. Serving both the sociological and anthropological constituencies at once means bridging ethnographic traditions, cultural foci, and socio-ecological approaches to embodiment and sensuousness. *The Senses in Self, Society, and Culture* is intended to be a milestone in the social sciences' somatic turn.

Phillip Vannini is Professor in the School of Communication and Culture at Royal Roads University, Victoria, Canada, and Canada Research Chair in Innovative Learning and Public Ethnography. He is author and editor of eight books, including *Understanding Society through Popular Music, Second Edition* (with Kotarba, Merrill, and Williams, 2013, Routledge), and *Ferry Tales: An Ethnography of Mobilities, Place, and Time on Canada's West Coast* (2011, Routledge).

Dennis Waskul is Professor of Sociology at Minnesota State University, Mankato. He is author of *Self-Games and Body-Play* (2003, Peter Lang), production editor for *Symbolic Interaction*, editor of *net.seXXX* (2004, Peter Lang), and co-editor of *Body/Embodiment* (2006, Ashgate). He has published numerous studies on the sociology of the body, senses, sexualities, and computer-mediated communications.

Simon Gottschalk is Associate Professor of Sociology at the University of Nevada, Las Vegas. He was editor of *Symbolic Interaction* (2003–2007), and is the author of numerous articles and book chapters on self-environment relations, postmodern culture, social psychology, qualitative research, the mass media, and interaction in virtual environments.

Contemporary Sociological Perspectives

Edited by **Doug Hartmann**, University of Minnesota, **Valerie Jenness**, University of California, Irvine and **Jodi O'Brien**, Seattle University

This innovative series is for all readers interested in books that provide frameworks for making sense of the complexities of contemporary social life. Each of the books in this series uses a sociological lens to provide current critical and analytical perspectives on significant social issues, patterns and trends. The series consists of books that integrate the best ideas in sociological thought with an aim toward public education and engagement. These books are designed for use in the classroom as well as for scholars and socially curious general readers.

Published:

Political Justice and Religious Values by Charles F. Andrain

GIS and Spatial Analysis for the Social Sciences by Robert Nash Parker and Emily K. Asencio

Hoop Dreams on Wheels: Disability and the Competitive Wheelchair Athlete by Ronald J. Berger

The Internet and Social Inequalities by James C. Witte and Susan E. Mannon

Media and Middle Class Mom: Images and Realities of Work and Family by Lara Descartes and Conrad Kottak

Watching T.V. Is Not Required: Thinking about Media and Thinking about Thinking by Bernard McGrane and John Gunderson

Violence Against Women: Vulnerable Populations by Douglas Brownridge

State of Sex: Tourism, Sex and Sin in the New American Heartland by Barbara G. Brents, Crystal A. Jackson & Kate Hausbeck

Social Statistics: The Basics and Beyond by Thomas J. Linneman

Sociologists Backstage: Answers to 10 Questions About What They Do by Sarah Fenstermaker and Nikki Jones

Gender Circuits by Eve Shapiro

Surviving the Holocaust: A Life Course Perspective by Ronald Berger

Transforming Scholarship: Why Women's and Gender Studies Students Are Changing Themselves and the World by Michelle Berger and Cheryl Radeloff

Stargazing: Celebrity, Fame, and Social Interaction by Kerry Ferris and Scott Harris

The Senses in Self, Society, and Culture by Phillip Vannini, Dennis Waskul and Simon Gottschalk

Who Lives, Who Dies, Who Decides? by Sheldon Ekland-Olson

Surviving Dictatorship by Jacqueline Adams

The Womanist Idea by Layli Maparyan

Social Theory Re-Wired: New Connections to Classical and Contemporary Perspectives by Wesley Longhofer and Daniel Winchester

Religion in Today's World: Global Issues, Sociological Perspectives by Melissa Wilcox

Life and Death Decisions: The Quest for Morality and Justice in Human Societies by Sheldon Ekland-Olson

Understanding Deviance: Connecting Classical and Contemporary Perspectives by Tammy L. Anderson

TITLES OF RELATED INTEREST:

The Connected City by Zachary Neal

Regression Analysis for the Social Sciences by Rachel A Gordon

Applied Statistics for the Social and Health Sciences by Rachel A Gordon

GIS and Spatial Analysis: A Tool for the Social Sciences by Robert Parker and Emily Asencio

THE SENSES IN SELF, SOCIETY, AND CULTURE

A Sociology of the Senses

Phillip Vannini, Dennis Waskul,
and Simon Gottschalk

Routledge
Taylor & Francis Group
NEW YORK AND LONDON

First published in paperback in 2014

First published 2012
by Routledge
711 Third Avenue, New York, NY 10017

and by Routledge
2 Park Square, Milton Park, Abingdon, Oxon OX14 4RN

Routledge is an imprint of the Taylor & Francis Group, an informa business

Library of Congress Cataloging-in-Publication Data
Vannini, Phillip.
The senses in self, society, and culture : a sociology of the senses / Phillip Vannini, Dennis Waskul, Simon Gottschalk
p. cm. — (Contemporary sociological perspectives)
Includes bibliographical references.
1.Senses and sensation—Social aspects. 2. Ethnopsychology.
I. Waskul, Dennis D., 1969– II. Gottschalk, Simon. III. Title.
BF233.V36 2011
302'.1—dc22 2011008517

ISBN 13: 978–0–415–87991–0 (hbk)
ISBN 13: 978–0–415–73104–1 (pbk)
ISBN 13: 978–0–203–80598–5 (ebk)

Typeset in Abode Caslon
by Keystroke, Station Road, Codsall, Wolverhampton

CONTENTS

SERIES EDITORS' FOREWORD

This innovative series is for all readers interested in books that provide frameworks for making sense of the complexities of contemporary social life. Each of the books in this series uses a sociological lens to provide current critical and analytical perspectives on significant social issues, patterns, and trends. The series consists of books that integrate the best ideas in sociological thought with an aim toward public education and engagement. These books are designed for use in the classroom as well as for scholars and socially curious general readers.

The Senses in Self, Society, and Culture contributes to a newly emerging literature on the connections between the body, mind, and culture. Most people assume their sensory responses are automatic and purely physical, but recent studies in the cultural processes of physical experience teach us that our responses are more complex than we realize. In this breakthrough book, Phillip Vannini, Dennis Waskul, and Simon Gottschalk identify the social processes that shape the seemingly physical responses associated with the five senses. Using empirical studies and provocative everyday examples, the authors illustrate the social construction of sensory experience. The book is ideal for anyone interested in sensory experiences such as "acquired taste" for specific foods, shifting changes in color preferences for fashion, smell memories, or cultural concepts of hygiene and odor.

Valerie Jenness and Jodi O'Brien
Series Editors

PREFACE AND ACKNOWLEDGMENTS

Fueled by the cultural and the bodily turn, for the last decade the social sciences have been witnessing a rapid growth of new subfields of study, such as the sociology and anthropology of the body and of the senses. Whereas the study of the body has enjoyed tremendous growth over the past decades and has perhaps by now reached maturity, the study of the senses is only recently coming into its own with the recent (2006) publication of the peer-reviewed journal *The Senses and Society*, the production of a few interdisciplinary readers, and the publication of a handful of foundational scholarly essays and monographs. Still absent, however, is a focused and comprehensive book that works as a map to the field and as the engine for further intellectual growth. Combining a thorough review of classical, recent, and emerging scholarship with grounded original empirical material as a strategy for sparking interest and deepening review and analysis, this book intends to be a key reference tool.

In contrast to books that separate the five (or six, or seven) senses from one another, our book is divided alongside points of intersections with existing sociological and anthropological fields of study. In doing so, we intend to appeal to a wide variety of scholars and students who are interested in a particular field of study other than the senses and who are keen on exploring linkages. Therefore, both our review of the literature and utilization of our own original empirical material unfold as "bridge-crossing" endeavors. Furthermore, we put a premium not only on the senses as subject matter of our interest, but also on sensuousness as a paradigm. Thus, this book does not solely review the literature but also develops—whenever possible—embodied knowledge-making by sensuously evoking concrete instances from everyday life.

The integrating theme running throughout the book links the past, present, and future significance of the "sensory," "sensual," "sensuous," and/or "somatic turn" to sociological and anthropological scholarship *on* the senses and *through* the senses. In bridging cultural sciences such as qualitative sociology, social and cultural anthropology, human geography, and cultural studies we intend explicitly to blur boundaries that, in this field, are particularly porous in light of the qualitative, phenomenological, interpretive, and ethnographic scope of much research. Simultaneously, given our interest in developing a sociological approach to the study of the senses, we hope this book will put the *sociology of the senses* on the map for good. In sum, the present book has been written for a wide audience comprised of advanced undergraduate students, graduate students, and scholars who are either entirely new to the field or already familiar with it but not with its most recent developments. Because we have such a wide audience in mind, our approach is comprehensive and we have taken care to use the richest literature possible.

This book would not have been possible without the assistance and support of many people. Our gratitude goes to Royal Roads University (RRU), which has supported our research through internal grants that have paid for some of the fieldwork expenses, as well as for travel to conferences where our findings and ideas have been shared. Jodi O'Brien and Steve Rutter at Routledge provided us with advice, direction, and support. Guppy Ahluwalia-Lopez assisted with data collection, analysis, and writing. Portions of the research cited in this book were aided by the collaboration of various co-authors, including Janelle Wilson, Carol Rambo, Toby Ellis-Newstead, and Desiree Wiesen. Their input was priceless.

Phillip, Dennis, and Simon also wish to acknowledge the kind permissions received by the University of California Press, Berg Publishers, Ashgate Publishing, and SAGE to reproduce excerpts from the following publications: "Sound Acts: Elocution, Somatic Work, and the Performance of Sonic Alignment," *Journal of Contemporary Ethnography*, (2010) 39:328–353; "Toward a Sensuous Understanding of Material Culture: Representing and Performing Taste at Wine Festivals," *Qualitative Inquiry*, (2010) 16:378–396; "The Aroma of Recollection: Olfaction, Nostalgia, and the Shaping of the Sensuous Self," *The Senses and Society*, (2008) 4:5–22; "Smell, Odor, and Somatic Work: Sense-Making and Sensory Management," *Social Psychology Quarterly*, (2008) 71:53–71; "Women and Their Clitoris: Personal Discovery, Signification, and Use," *Symbolic Interaction*, (2007) 30:151–174; and "Paddle and Portage: The Travail of BWCA Canoe Travel," in P. Vannini (ed.) (2009), *The Cultures of Alternative Mobility: Routes Less Travelled*, 21–37.

Part I

Understanding Sensory Studies

1

TOWARD A SOCIOLOGY OF THE SENSES

Returning home from a doctor's appointment, I (Dennis) park my vehicle in the garage and enter my home through the rear porch. Nobody is home. Walking in the porch, I immediately smell a potent and toxic aroma that unleashes a flow of adrenalin, quickens my heartbeat, and accelerates my breathing. "Natural gas," I quickly decide. My four-year-old son has in the past managed to turn on the oven burners, causing them to belch deadly gas into our home. Bolting indoors, I immediately race to the stove to check whether it is the source of the noxious odor. Not this time. The oven and burners are off. I check to make sure the pilot lights are working properly. Yep. Everything seems normal. I continue to investigate my home and make my way toward the basement. Perhaps the pilot light on the furnace has gone out. Maybe the water heater? By now, the toxic odor has dissipated. I no longer smell anything unusual or out of the ordinary, but I am still anxious. For the next fifteen minutes, I find myself sniff-testing the various zones of my home. Something caused that odor. What was it?

I am pacing aimlessly about the house, still trying to trace the source of the odor. Along the way I notice that our dog has once again eaten all of the cat's food. Irritated with our fattening mutt, I grab the cat's tiny food dish and return to the back porch where we store the pet food. As I open the porch door, I am again assaulted by the toxic odor. This time, however, I notice something I previously missed: four large latex balloons that our children had purchased on a recent shopping trip. The day before, my wife and I needed a reprieve from their loud and rowdy playing with the balloons. Taking advantage of a moment when they were preoccupied with something else, we quickly and quietly moved the balloons into the back porch where they have since remained, and now the tiny enclosed porch is filled with the potent aroma of latex. Mystery solved. Relieved, I proceed with my usual activities.

What does smell indicate? How do we interpret its meaning? How does the perception of an odor that we do not expect or anticipate compel us to *make sense* of what we are sensing? How could I have mistaken the smell of latex for natural gas, and why did it bother me so? Perhaps because I perceive that same antiseptic latex aroma in hospitals and doctors' offices, from whence I had just returned, and it is a smell I dislike because I associate it with bad memories. Perhaps it is because my son in the past has turned on the burners on the stove and left them on. In either case, how does memory inform sensory perception? What if I were not alone during this moment of olfactory uncertainty—what if my wife were home? I have no doubt the dialogue would be something like this:

"Honey, what's that smell?"

"I don't know. What smell?"

"Come over here. Can't you smell it? It smells like gas."

[Sniff-sniff, sniff-sniff] "Oh, I smell it now. Smells more like rubber to me."

And the conversation would carry on until we mutually agreed on a common somatic definition of the situation—or gave up trying altogether. Why was it so important for me to identify that odor? Why did I even notice it in the first place? After all, the balloons had been in our home for several days, and I had not noticed the odor before. Clearly, many biographical, contextual, social, and cultural factors entered my sense-making practices that, until moments like these, are barely noticeable. Perhaps, as anthropologist Paul Stoller illustrates, the same may be said of *all* sensory experience.

Few scholars have more passionately called for a heightened awareness and appreciation of the senses than Paul Stoller. His vision of a "sensuous awakening" closely approximates our ambitions in this book. The challenge, according to Stoller, is twofold. First, scholars need to learn to rediscover the deep significance of sensations. This may require re-learning to sense, especially in environments that are foreign to a researcher. Second, scholars need to present sensations in evocative, passionate, carnal, and imaginative ways. This may require experimenting with writing, with organization of one's work, and with different modes of representation (e.g. film, performing arts, etc.):

> Stiffened from long sleep in the background of scholarly life, the scholar's body yearns to exercise its muscles. Sleepy from long inactivity, it aches to restore its sensibilities. Adrift in a sea of half-lives, it wants to breathe in the pungent odors of social life, to run its palms over the jagged surface of social reality, to hear the wondrous symphonies of social experience, to see the sensuous shapes and colors that fill windows of consciousness. It wants to awaken the imagination and bring scholarship back to "the

things themselves." Wants, however, are far from being deeds, for a sensuous awakening is a very tall order in an academy where mind has long been separated from the body, sense long revered from sensibility. This scholarly disconnectedness is the very antithesis of Mojud's sensuous celebrations of life. What can his embodied example mean to *fin de siècle* scholars?

(Stoller 1997:xii)

THE SOCIAL SENSES

It would appear that "the five senses" are a matter of common sense, and yet few experiences are more socially constructed. The fact that we may see, hear, smell, taste, and feel through touch makes it, perhaps, all too difficult to recognize that we experience these sensations in ways that are much more "contaminated" than they appear to be. For example, every morning I enjoy a cup or two of strong coffee—and not only for a caffeinated jolt to my groggy mind. I genuinely enjoy the total sensual experience of fresh-brewed morning coffee. The taste of coffee incorporates its smell, but the smell of the coffee I drink is quite different from the tantalizing aroma of brewing coffee, a scent that, in fact, seems to awaken my senses. Even though the two aromas are different, I know that the smell of brewing coffee anticipates and lubricates how I both taste and smell coffee when I drink it. When I am traveling, a morning cup of coffee is not nearly so satisfying. This is partly because, at a restaurant or gas station, I am usually not seduced by the aroma of the brewing process.

The flavor of coffee also includes the feel of hot liquid. In the morning, it has to be hot. I occasionally enjoy iced-coffee, but iced-coffee would never satisfy me in the morning, regardless of environmental temperature. Even the weight and feel of the mug are significant. I find it hard to get a satisfying swig from those dainty, undersized, bourgeois, espresso cups. Conversely, if the mug is too large the coffee is cold before I'm finished. Glass mugs are cute, but they hopelessly fail to insulate and quickly become scalding hot to grasp with my hands. I prefer a mid-size, thick ceramic mug.

The taste, the smell, the tactile feel of coffee in the morning—all these sensations blend into a total sensual experience in which the whole is greater than the sum of its parts.

As we will see in Chapter 3, the same can be said of wine connoisseurs, and we can all recognize these same kinds of total sensual experience in our lives—those moments of multi-sensuality when the experience of one sense cannot be separated from others. Moreover, these experiences are not exactly synesthesia-like either; we merely experience "the five senses" in ways that are not as discrete as "common sense" seems to imply. In fact, in most circumstances, when I seek to specify a sensual experience, I am rarely able to pin it entirely on one mode of sensing. Can you? Can anyone? Indeed, if it were possible to characterize sensations and feelings precisely, would poetry continue to exist? Would language not work more like math? Would all of the arts not feel like positive sciences?

To suggest that the senses are socially constructed is not an excuse for yet again invoking an old metaphor. After all, most social scientists agree that, regardless of what it may be, their topic of interest is subject to social construction, negotiation, regulation, and control. Rather, the claim that the senses are constructions suggests that they are not passive receptors, and that sensations are not the passive objects of those receptors. By claiming that they are constructions, we highlight their quality as products and practice, as action and interaction, as work and performance. Whether the senses are constructed by sensory orders that stipulate which sensory domain is more "important" (e.g. Classen 1993, 1998), whether sensations are actively sought by hedonistic wine drinkers in search of the perfect taste (e.g. Hennion 2007), or whether sensual cultures are built through rituals that stipulate somatic rules and sensuous performances (e.g. Stoller 1989), the human senses and sensations are certainly the subject matter of cultural and social scientists, and not the sole domain of physiology and cognition.

Furthermore, the very notion that there are *five* senses is purely arbitrary (see Classen 1993; Geurts 2003). Why only five? If we wished to, we could identify at least eight, and perhaps divide them into two categories. The taken-for-granted five senses belong to those sensory modes that provide information about the world *external* to us. Those are our exteroceptive senses: sight, hearing, taste, smell, and touch. It is easy enough to identify at least three more senses that provide information about the *internal* world of the human body, our interoceptive senses: the sense of pain (nociception), thirst, and hunger. Yet, eight is not nearly enough. What about our sense of our own internal muscles and organs (proprioception)? What about the sensations that mediate between conditions in the external world and internal body, such as our sense of balance (equilibrioception), movement (kinesthesia), temperature (thermoception), or even our sense of time (at least in terms of polychronicity and monochronicity, if not more)? Now our list has grown from five senses to thirteen, and still we experience senses that are not clearly accounted for in these categories. After all, which category accounts for the sensual experience of orgasm? Assuming one can come up with an answer, which is doubtful, it is unlikely that we would agree—especially considering that even within the experiences of one individual, not all orgasms are the same.

We may even suggest that to divide the senses into categories is itself an arbitrary act that reproduces our cultural frames of reference. In fact, why divide "external" from "internal" senses at all? Is doing so not an exercise in dualism, atomism, and individualism so typical of Western culture? And because understanding most of our sensations, and thus our senses, depends so heavily on the language that we use (Geurts 2003), should we not treat the senses in their own cultural contexts and within "their own foundational schemas through which the world is . . . sensed as a continuous whole" (Edwards, Gosden, and Phillips 2006:6)? And finally, are we even certain that sensations can be so clearly separated from emotions, or even from the material stimuli that are the object of sensations (see Geurts 2003; Ingold 2000; Thrift 2008)? What we do know for sure is that to think of the senses as only confined to five exteroceptive sensory modes is grossly to oversimplify human sensual experience, both within and across cultures. Maybe that is the key point: modes of sensing inevitably blend and blur into one another, thus making their alleged boundaries fuzzy and indistinct in experience. It is this ecology of affective relations that should be the focus of our attention (see Howes 2003; Ingold 2000; Thrift 2008).

Conversely, the codes we rely on to classify sensory experience are mutable into seemingly infinite ways that socially and culturally carve out what Zerubavel (1991) called "islands of meaning." It is, in fact, those islands of meaning that largely (but not entirely) make sensory experience perceptible, namely by transforming them into arbitrary yet significant symbols (Mead 1934). As Zerubavel (1996) argued, the worlds in which we live are essentially continuous, yet we experience them in discrete chunks. This is especially true of the ever-discerning sensual body and the ever-selective nature of sensual experience. We understand, and indeed make sense out of, sensory experience by creating distinct mental clusters through processes that Zerubavel (1996) calls "lumping" and "splitting." Lumping "entails grouping 'similar' things together in a single mental cluster," while splitting "involves perceiving 'different' clusters as separate from one another" (Zerubavel 1996:421). While the processes of lumping and splitting may seem "natural," they actively construct significant distinctions that, once acquired (most often through linguistic constructs), we treat "as if they were part of nature" because "we have been socialized to 'see' them" (Zerubavel 1996:426–427). For example, as Zerubavel points out, it is by sheer convention that we perceive grape juice as similar to orange juice, and dissimilar from wine. This distinction has little to do with the taste of either wine or grape juice; instead, it has everything to do with a cultural process of lumping that is made possible by the splitting construct of "alcohol." The concept of alcohol, not the sensory experience of the drink, leads us to perceive wine as more similar to whisky than to grape juice. Yet, without the ability to lump and split, it is impossible to envision any mental cluster at all (Zerubavel 1996). While the mind organizes reality into separate chunks, we do not do this as individuals, but as members of social and cultural "thought communities" (Zerubavel 1996), and, extrapolating from Zerubavel, as members of social and cultural *sensory communities*: groups of people who share common ways of using their senses and making sense of sensations.

There are countless ways in which the human senses are subject to the reach of sensory communities across cultures and societies. For example, our individual and collective memories include what we eat and drink, how food and beverages feel and taste, and how those people close to us are involved in tasting with us and establishing a sense of community around the foods we choose (Serematakis 1994). The taste of prepared food—whether a recipe is well or poorly prepared, lavishly or modestly made—is also the subject of social norms, roles, and scripts that are passed down from generation to generation and observed in specific circumstances of commensality (Choo 2004; Stoller 1989; Sutton 2001). Sensory communities' aesthetic preferences with regard to specific sensations also inform the norms that regulate self-presentation, such as those that stipulate how one's body should smell (Classen 1992; Largey and Watson 1972; Waskul and Vannini 2008) and how the bodies of people of different ethnicities are expected to smell or not to smell (Low 2005, 2006). Sensory communities are also involved in constructing "sensory rituals" (Howes 1987), ranging from meals at the family table (Sutton 2001) to the soundscapes that make places meaningful (Feld 1982; Feld and Basso 1996; Jackson 1968; Panopoulos 2003), and from the mundane experience of commuting (Edensor 2003) to the experience of illness (Chuengsatiansup 1999), healing (Desjarlais 2003), and healthy bodily movement (Sparkes 2009). The list could go on endlessly, but the point is that the senses are the "most fundamental domain of cultural expression, the medium through which all of the values and practices are enacted" (Howes 2003:xi), "part of the set of physiologically grounded human skills which render a world intelligible and workable" (Edwards, Gosden, and Phillips 2006:5), and thus the very basis of human experience and interaction (Dewey 1934; Merleau-Ponty 1962; Serres 2008).

THE PURPOSE OF THIS BOOK

In our everyday lives, most of us pay little conscious attention to *how* we sense. To be sure, as the opening paragraphs of this introduction show, we do pay a great deal of attention to *what* we sense, but the *ways* in which we sense most often recede into the background of our awareness. As Leder (1990) has observed, most of our routine bodily experience is marked by lack of reflection, and it is only when routines and habits are interrupted—for example, when we suddenly feel sick, or when a sensation overwhelms us—that our own sensual experience "awakens" our embodied consciousness. In light of this lack of attention, most of us have become accustomed to think of our senses as neutral media that, when they work properly, perform like conduits of external stimuli. Take this book, for example. The texture, color, shape, and size of the pages that you are holding seem to be nothing but rather elementary stimuli that your senses of sight and touch "transmit"—much like information bits—to your brain for processing. There seems to be very little *social* significance whatsoever in this process, doesn't there? Perhaps this is why, after all, most people view perception as a rather cognitive affair and sensation as a purely physiological one.

The purpose of this book is to transcend models of human sensation and perception—such as the one based on transmission and processing that was summarily sketched out above—that are based on a dualist ontology. Grounded in binary oppositions, dualist ontology often separates mind from body (Williams and Bendelow 1998). In this perspective, the mind is a tool that processes raw information furnished by the body's physiological organs into complex cognitive matter. As one can glean from this model, not only are the body and the mind separate and distinct from one another, but so are (raw) sensations and (cognitive) perceptions, and so are the individuals and the objective worlds in which stimuli occur. Dualisms of this kind—and many others could be identified—are gross simplifications of a complex and emergent ecological system that is, fortunately, much more interesting than such predictability-based models propose. By refusing to separate sensation from perception, the body from the mind, and the individual from "external stimuli," our approach to senses and sensations advances a post-dualist and post-representational ontology (e.g. Thrift 2008) that, since Dewey's (1934) classic work on experience, has progressively swept across the social sciences. In doing so we posit an approach to senses and sensations that is thoroughly *social.*

We are not the first to suggest that the human senses and sensations are of social significance. As we will detail in the following section, many anthropologists have been aware of the deeply significant cultural dimensions of the senses for at least two decades, and so have some philosophers (e.g. Lingis 1996; Merleau-Ponty 1962; Serres 2008) historians (e.g. Harvey 2006; Hoffer 2003; Smith 2007), business managers and designers (e.g. Lindstrom 2005; Malnar and Vodvarka 2004), geographers (e.g. Adams and Guy 2007; Rodaway 1994), psychologists (e.g. Gibson 1983), communication scholars (e.g. Banes and Lepecki 2006; Bull and Back 2003; Finnegan 2002; Ong 1982), and sociologists (e.g. Fine 1995; Low 2006; Synnott 1993). Yet, the existing scholarship of the senses seems to lack a comprehensive bridge between narrow research interests and analytical reflection. Thus, for example, while students and scholars interested in research on smell (e.g. Drobnick 2006), sight (e.g. Edwards and Bhaumik 2008), hearing (e.g. Bull and Back 2003), touch (e.g. Classen 2005), taste (e.g. Korsmeyer 2005), or even the "sixth sense" (e.g. Howes 2009) are now able to access the scholarship on the particular sense that interests them, anyone interested in a more global, comprehensive, and foundational approach to the social aspects of the human senses, sensations, and sense-making writ large would have a difficult time locating helpful resources.

While claims to academic inter- and trans-disciplinarity abound these days, few of these are realized in practice. Therefore, any attempt to cross disciplinary boundaries, such as ours, must first be qualified and then exercised with caution. The three of us are trained in sociology; two of us (Dennis and Simon) make their livings in sociology departments, and the third (Phillip) works in a school of communication and culture. While our published research has spanned media studies, cultural studies, communication studies, human geography, and social anthropology, most of our publications are of a sociological nature (broadly defined). Moreover, the three of us have strong affiliations with symbolic interactionism—a classical sociological perspective, albeit a rather interdisciplinary one. In sum, while it would be tempting to claim to offer a foundational book in the transdisciplinary field of "sensory studies," it is much more prudent and realistic to focus our efforts on a "sociology of the senses" that is not parochial (as mainstream sociology can be) but rather fully inclusive of all the cultural sciences. Indeed, this is a field that some might call a natural blend of cultural sociology and social anthropology.

We feel that the blurring of the boundaries between sociology and anthropology is natural enough to cause little anxiety among our most theoretically conservative readers, and adventurous enough to motivate our more progressive audiences to join us on a post-disciplinary ride that liberally hops between and across communication studies, human geography, and cultural studies, as well as, of course, sociology and anthropology. Indeed, as we detail in later chapters, the key conceptual purpose of our book is to lay out the analytical foundations for an approach to *the senses as interaction*. In positing the senses as interaction we open up the field to anyone—regardless of disciplinary affiliation—keen to understand sensuality as sociality, and human experiences as sensuousness. In light of the above, we promote both a subject matter and a particular approach, rather than the state of art of a particular sub-discipline.

THE HISTORICAL EVOLUTION OF THE SOCIOLOGICAL AND ANTHROPOLOGICAL STUDY OF THE SENSES

Attempts to outline the scope and history of the anthropology of the senses may be very recent, but they are certainly no longer new. Starting with David Howes's edited volume *The Varieties of Sensory Experience* (1991) anthropologists have periodically reflected on the development of this growing field within their discipline through anthologies of previously collected materials (e.g. Howes 2005 and the "Sensory Formations" series published by Berg), methodological reflections (e.g. Pink 2006; Stoller 1997), theoretical interventions (e.g. Howes 2003) and special issues of various journals (e.g. *Ethnos* 2008(4) and *Etnofoor* 2007(1); and, outside anthropology, see *Culture and Organization* 2006(3) and *Journal of Social History* 2007(summer)). Useful historical material pertinent to anthropology and related fields can also be found online at the newly formed sensorystudies.org website. The same cannot be said of sociologists of the senses, and it is with them that we start this brief overview of the field.

Like other academics, sociologists tend to feel that a new sub-discipline has taken a firm hold when a new study group or section is established within one of their major professional associations. Since the American Sociological Association, the British Sociological Association, the International Sociological Association, and the European Sociological Association have yet to see the birth of a group dedicated to the study of the senses, one wonders whether sociology as a whole is less prepared to address the theoretical and methodological questions raised by students of the senses. If the existence of a section within a major professional organization seems like too stringent a criterion, however, perhaps other criteria ought to be considered. Coalitions based on sub-disciplinary interest may form, for example, around university departments with a particular research and teaching emphasis, small research networks either standing on their own feet or built around minor professional organizations, or around periodic thematic conferences. But on the basis of these criteria, too, one would be hard pressed to find a sociology of the senses as a clearly recognizable and full-standing substantive sub-field such as, for example, the sociology of the body is today. At this point our readers might wonder whether we, as the authors of this book, should even dedicate our attention to a field so new that it barely even exists. In spite of its appearance, however, the sociology of the senses is not too far behind the anthropology of the senses. Furthermore, we believe that combining the sociology and the anthropology of the senses will foster the progress of both.

So, is there a sociology of the senses at all, given what we have just said? Our answer is "yes." The sociology of the senses is rooted in the classical social theory of Georg Simmel, George Herbert Mead, William James, and especially John Dewey. Simmel's essays on sociological aesthetics, the sociology of the meal, and the senses themselves (Simmel 1997) show how sociologists can gain a better understanding of social relations by extending aesthetic categories to forms of society (see De la Fuente 2007). On the other hand, American pragmatist philosophers, such as Mead, Dewey, and James, show throughout their scholarship how sensing is an active and interpretive process, rather than a passive reaction to external stimuli endowed with pre-formed meaning. It is in Mead's (1938) philosophy of the act, Dewey's (1934) anti-dualist understanding of experience as a form of aesthetic transaction between the individual and its world, and James's (1983) psychology of emotions that one can find the genesis of a sociological theory of the senses. In addition to these often-quoted founders of symbolic interaction theory, a sociology of the senses is rooted in the phenomenological writings of Maurice Merleau-Ponty (1962) on the embodiment of perception and social existence.

This very early period of interest in what today can be defined as a crypto-sociology of the senses was later developed by such interactionists as Becker and Goffman. While neither can be pegged as a sociologist of the senses, both of these founding fathers of modern sociology inspired the contemporary interest in a sociology of the senses. Becker's essays on jazz (1951) and marijuana-smoking (1963), for example, show that hearing and taste are subject to processes of socialization, cultivation, and interpersonal regulation, and therefore that sensations function much like embodied skills and techniques. Goffman's attention to the visual aspects of interaction, notable throughout his entire oeuvre, culminated in his book *Gender Advertisements* (1979): a visual examination of how gender scripts and related visual props enable the performance of gendered bodies. This period of uneven attention to the sensory components of interaction in Western society (1950s through 1970s) was also marked by the publication of thought-provoking but sporadic studies, such as Largey and Watson's (1972) piece on the sociology of smell.

It was not until the 1990s that sociologists on both sides of the Atlantic became more comfortable with novel topics, such as the sociology of the body, and later the sociology of the senses (e.g. Synnott 1993). Ushered in by postmodern theory, post-structuralism, and cultural studies, the cultural turn of the 1980s further solidified, if not legitimized, various forms of non-positivist sociology. The emergence of new discourses prompted the rapid growth of such fields as the sociology of culture, of gender, of the emotions, of food, of music, of the arts, of popular culture and the media, and the rapid institutionalization of such qualitative research traditions as interpretive ethnography and visual methodology. At the same time, this turn also allowed for the renewal of interest in qualitative social psychological perspectives, such as those represented by various strands of symbolic interactionism. As sociology became less uneasy about its macro versus micro, quantitative versus qualitative, and structure versus agency divisions, qualitative sociologists like Fine quickly gained prominence with sense-related ethnographic studies of chefs (1996) and mushroom pickers (2003). At the same time, Howard Becker's (2000) call to embrace a visual sociology and Norman Denzin's manifestos (e.g. 1996) for a reflexive, narrative, and post-realist epistemology further blurred the boundaries between traditional scientific writing and a more sensuous, or at least sensitive and embodied, sociological enterprise. Importantly, in 1993, Anthony Synnott published a monograph that laid the foundations for a historic-sociological approach to the senses as an extension of the then nascent sociological interest in the body in general.

As the sociology of the body continued to grow throughout the 1990s and the early years of the new millennium, however, ever more of the early "embodied turn" dissolved into a sociology that treated the body as a sign divorced from its lived experience. While phenomenological investigations of lived bodies now exist in the literature, they are vastly outnumbered by other approaches that ignore the carnal sensations of actual human beings and their embodied relations with others. Most of these are deconstructions of the codes that regulate the body's semiotic meanings, critical macro-examinations of the "body social," and philosophical speculations on "the" body—understood in abstraction from its experience and environment. A sociology of the senses must thus be understood as a reaction to the theoretical excesses of a sociology of the body that morphed the body from an absent presence (cf. Shilling 1993) to a presence silenced by theoretical noise. A sociology of the senses therefore attempts, in large part, to rediscover humans' sensuous, erotic, and aesthetic transactions with one another and their environments.

While the last few years have certainly seen the emergence of a coherent sociological approach to the senses, the terrain is far from smooth. For instance, the social study of the senses is a field that has grown more rapidly in the United Kingdom (where the boundaries between social anthropology and cultural sociology have long been very loosely drawn) than in North America, where cultural anthropology and qualitative sociology have long shared a methodology—ethnography—while blissfully ignoring each other. Furthermore, as mentioned above, the absence of a founding text capable of bridging disciplinary divisions has prevented the building of a unified front.

Writing from North America puts us in an interesting position from which to advocate a sociological approach to the senses. While we are somewhat removed from the few loose and informal groups that have coalesced around this topic in the UK, it is in North America that recent advances in ethnographic methodology and interpretive social psychological and sociocultural perspectives, such as symbolic interactionism and performance theory, have a deeper hold. Of course, we do not intend to generate Balkanizing continental divisions by stating this. Rather, we agree with the editors of the field's own journal—*The Senses and Society*, first published in 2006—that sociology has a key role to play in further blurring continental and disciplinary boundaries. And the key step in doing so is by building upon the contributions of the anthropology of the senses, while striving to fill its gaps.

The Anthropology of the Senses

Whereas a sociology of the senses is at best in its infancy, an anthropology of the senses has almost reached maturity. Since David Howes (2003) has carefully outlined the intellectual development of the anthropology of the senses, it is best to avoid repetitions of that work and only briefly summarize it here. According to Howes, anthropologists have always had a latent interest in the senses. At first this interest manifested itself in classification hierarchies, such as those between the visual cultures of the West—believed to be superior, as sight was taken to be a more objective mode of perception of the world—and the more "animal-like" sensory cultures of the rest of the world. An examination of early anthropological texts shows that the sensory acuity of non-white ethnic groups' experiences of touch, taste, and smell were particularly denigrated for their properties of overwhelming emotionality, "brute" corporeality, and the need for copresence, in contrast to the cognitive and abstract power afforded by the "distant" senses of sight and hearing (see Synnott 1993).

As early, often deeply racist, anthropological interest classification and ranking subsided, anthropologists' concern with the senses shifted to an interest in sensations as texts. This movement was, of course, attributable to the tremendous influence of Clifford Geertz's (1973) fieldwork in Bali. Geertz's hermeneutic and semiotic approach to culture treated experience as a text to be read in accordance with rules and codes operating in a particular situation and context. His symbolic anthropology was distinct from the other highly popular theoretical perspective of the time—Levi-Straussian structuralism—but to some degree it replicated structuralism's overriding concern with deciphering the systems of symbols on which cultures are believed to be based. As Csordas (1993) would later insightfully observe, much of both structuralism and symbolic anthropology tend to overemphasize cognitive and abstract meaning at the expense of the carnality and the practical value of bodily experience. However, the influence of Csordas's powerful critique was not to be felt until the beginning of the new millennium, since, as Howes (2003) observed, so much anthropology in the 1990s was concerned with struggles over the politics of ethnographic representation, the authority of texts, and reflexivity.

Howes's treatment of the postmodern turn in ethnographic writing is a skeptical and even critical one. For him, the quest for reflexivity that marked ethnographic writing after the publication of Clifford and Marcus's (1986) influential edited volume constituted more of a distraction than anything else. As he saw it, the seemingly endless and vexing existential crisis of 1990s anthropology was most clearly visible in Stephen Tyler's (1986:137) claim that "perception has nothing to do" with ethnographic writing. But whereas Howes views Tyler's claim as a sign of the decadence of ethnography into empty aestheticism, other anthropologists, such as Stoller (see 1997), view the reflexive turn in ethnography as an opportunity to establish a sensuous scholarship that depends on the researcher's embodied presence in the field, and thus his/her ability to experiment with modes of representation that evoke sensuality, rather than just treat the senses as objects of analytical scrutiny. To assert that perception has nothing to do with ethnographic writing is undoubtedly a mistake; this assertion opens the door for an epistemology that is no longer framed by the principle of one "true" objective perception, but rather is informed by a post-realist mode where a *multitude of perceptions* enriches the diverse forms, objects, and genres of ethnographic knowledge.

At present, it is unclear where the anthropology of the senses is heading. Two directions can be identified: one dangerous; the other infinitely more promising. The first direction is disciplinary insularity. While human geography, cultural studies, and communication studies scholars have fully embraced a post-disciplinary and post-realist orientation, too many anthropologists see the study of the senses as existing in isolation from developments "outside" of their discipline. As a result, this body of research risks stagnation and a hypostasis of "the senses" (or, worse yet, one sense at a time), much like what has happened to the study of "the body." The second trend is much rosier. A growing volume of anthropological research has begun to experiment with new theoretical, conceptual, substantive, methodological, and disciplinary fusions, and has thus pushed for new epistemologies and ontologies that are less based on linguistic cognition and more on embodied, multi-sensual, multimodal, pre-objective, and carnal ways of knowing.

Since we feel that neither sociology alone nor anthropology alone—nor, for that matter, any other discipline, whether traditional or not—can fruitfully undertake the study of the senses and of sensations in all its complexity, we wish to offer in this book a perspective that is truly ecumenical, rather than reproducing tired orthodoxies. Whether one studies the senses and sensation from the viewpoint of geographical space, historical time, technological medium, culture, social structure, or the individual, we understand the senses and sensations as the lifeblood of embodied sociality and materiality, as the very tools and techniques allowing for the transaction between human and non-human agents, and the very condition for the carnal experience of selfhood, society, and culture. Of course, we are not under the illusion that any perspective can be broad enough to accommodate everyone, regardless of interest or philosophical orientation. However, in beginning our conceptual exercise by positing the senses and sensations as the key form of humans' active construction of the world, we hope to appeal to as broad a spectrum as possible. We find the metaphor of *work* especially useful to understand the senses, so it is to the treatment of somatic work that we now turn.

OUR THEORETICAL APPROACH: SOMATIC WORK

> [S]ensory experiences are produced, enacted and perceived in combination with each other, intertwined with emotion, meaning and memory.
>
> (Hsu 2008:440)

The basic premise of this book can be stated as follows: *humans sense as well as make sense*. This process of sense-making entails minded and embodied social and cultural practices that cannot be explained or reduced to physiological processes alone. The senses "are fundamental to personhood" and they concern "bodily engagement with the world," thus creating a structure "both offering and constraining possibilities for the human subject" (Edwards, Gosden, and Phillips 2006:23). They mediate between meaning and materiality—"sensory experience is socially made and mediated" (Hsu 2008:433)—and they "mediate the relationship between self and society, mind and body, idea and object" (Bull, Gilroy, Howes, and Kahn 2006:5). The senses are skills (Ingold 2000) that we actively employ in interpreting and evaluating the world. To see, for example, entails more than opening our eyes to allow light passively to bounce off our retinas. We must actively perceive that which is seen and thus *make sense* of somatic experience (see Howes 2003; Rodaway 1994). In this way, sensing and sense-making are necessarily conjoined, codetermined, and mutually emergent in active and reflexive practices in which we are both the subject and object of the sensations we perceive or, for that matter, fail to recognize. Take, for example, the image overleaf.

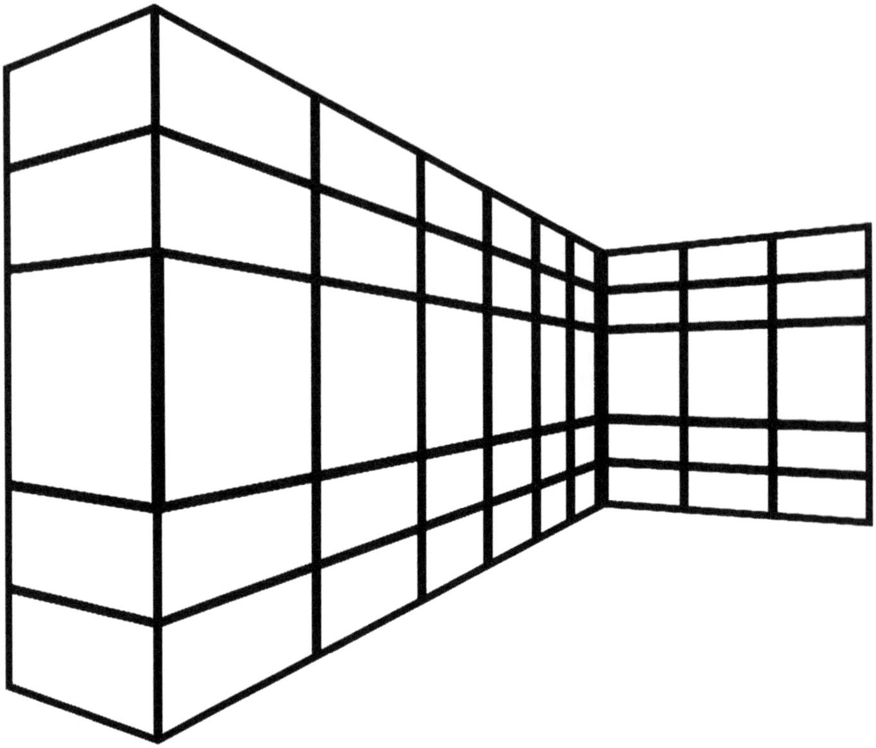

As René Descartes (2010:12) famously wrote, "the senses deceive from time to time, and it is a mark of prudence never to place our complete trust in those who have deceived us even once." Indeed, things are not always what they seem: in the image above, the bold line on the left is the same length as the bold line on the right, yet the sense-making practices we use to interpret what we see makes the line on the right appear much longer—an illusion produced by how we interpret visual sensory data, not what those data are. As this example illustrates, there is a difference between sensory modes and sensory codes (Stroeken 2008). The former emerge from the bodily stimulation of sense organs, while the latter are situational and socially shaped. Sensory perception is emergent between modes and codes. In the example above, how we code the two bold lines makes us perceive something that is not what it appears to be—perhaps like mistaking the aroma of latex for natural gas. Plainly stated, sense-making practices entail both creative and ritualized habits of the senses that draw from social, cultural, and semiotic resources by which we interpret and assign meaning to somatic awareness. As we explore in the pages that follow, these dynamics are complex, layered, and nuanced.

In his classic essay on the sociology of the senses Georg Simmel (1997: 109) suggested that the social sciences—sociology in particular—are "situated in this stage of being able to consider only the very large and clearly visible social structures and of trying to be able to produce insight from these into social life in its totality." Simmel does not necessarily question this macroscopic emphasis. He does, however, take issue with its rigidity. The central elements of social and cultural order are crystallized in "pulsating life which links human beings together" in embodied, sensual ways that connect individuals to social existence (Simmel 1997:109). So it is with the senses and sensory experience that "one's sociality, if not acquired and maintained through bodily experiences, finds bodily expression" (Hsu 2008:438). Indeed, sensual life pulsates with our individual and collective socio-cultural being so as to body forth our embodied self in time, space, and the symbolic worlds we occupy.

In attempting to flesh out these premises, this book seeks to explore how the senses are experiences that fit into a larger scheme. This larger cultural scheme is not necessarily "dependent on the unique characteristics of individual actors, but links the smallest social forces with the largest and the tiniest interaction arenas to the more expansive" (Fine and Hallett 2003:2).

Huxley's Lesson

Sense-making practices are largely produced in the process of what we call "somatic work." This refers to mundane, ritualized, and largely taken-for-granted practices. We will detail what we mean by somatic work in a moment, but as a narrative preface let us first illustrate it in the context of the lessons learned by Aldous Huxley. In *The Art of Seeing*, Huxley (1942:vii) narrates how, at the age of sixteen, he "had a violent attack of *keratitis punctata*." This, he writes, "left me (after eighteen months of near-blindness, during which I had to depend on Braille for my reading and a guide for my walking) with one eye just capable of light perception, and the other with enough vision to permit of my detecting the two-hundred foot letter on the Snellen chart at ten feet." For the next few years, doctors advised Huxley to read with the aid of a powerful hand-held magnifying glass—before later promoting him to spectacles—which allowed him "to read tolerably well—provided always that [he] kept [his] better pupil dilated with atropine, so that [he] might see round a particularly heavy patch of opacity at the center of the cornea" (Huxley 1942:vii). The task of reading caused Huxley considerable strain and fatigue, and when he finally acknowledged that his "capacity to see was steadily and quite rapidly failing," he discovered a method of visual re-education (Huxley 1942:viii). Within a few months, he was reading without spectacles—and without strain or fatigue. At last, the opacity in the cornea, "which had remained unchanged for upwards of twenty-five years, was beginning to clear up" (Huxley 1942:viii–ix). Although his vision was far from normal, Huxley had succeeded in teaching himself to see by re-educating his vision, and with a clarity of sight that was "about twice as good as it used to be when I wore spectacles" (Huxley 1942:ix).

Huxley's ability to re-educate his failing vision caused him to question how and why previous ophthalmological treatments had failed him so miserably. His conclusion was that ophthalmology has "been obsessively preoccupied with only one aspect of the total, complex process of seeing—the physiological. Ophthalmologists have paid attention exclusively to eyes, not at all to the mind which makes use of the eyes to see with" (Huxley 1942:x). For the balance of his book, Huxley offers scathing criticism of standard ophthalmology. He details techniques and practices for visual re-education by rejecting the facile assumption that vision is merely a passive product of properly functioning organs and by embracing the "art of seeing" as an active and minded process—something that we do in habitual yet creative ways (by which seeing is made to happen).

By the "art of seeing" Huxley (1942:35) means psycho-physical skills and habits that are typically "acquired in early infancy or childhood by a process of mainly unconscious self-instruction." In the case of vision, these habits of the senses entail "three subsidiary processes—a process of sensing, a process of selecting, and a process of perceiving" (Huxley 1942:42). Emphasizing that the last of these processes is necessarily reflexive, he concludes:

> sensing is not the same as perceiving. The eyes and nervous system do the sensing, the mind does the perceiving. The faculty of perceiving is related to the individual's accumulated experiences, in other words, to memory . . . Any improvement in the power of perceiving tends to be accompanied by an improvement in the power of sensing and of that product of sensing and perceiving which is seeing.
>
> (Huxley 1942:42)

Even though Huxley's language is clearly dualist, his "art of seeing" is one application of what we have more generally coined "somatic work"—the often taken-for-granted, if not transparent, practices of sense-making. While Huxley would discover what we call somatic work as a means for restoring his vision, we *all*—as individuals, as groups, as societies, and as cultures—routinely engage in forms of somatic work as part of the everyday life worlds we inhabit.

Somatic Work: Sensual Reflexivity, Transaction, and the Senses

> sen-sa-tion: *n.* 1. A perception associated with stimulation of a sense organ or with a specific body condition. 2. The faculty to feel or perceive.

By definition, sensation implies transaction: to sense is to *perceive* and the act of perception necessitates the *faculty to* feel or perceive. In other words, sensation (noun) is emergent in acts of sensing (verb). Senses and sensations are emergent in a relationship between specific modes of touch, smell, taste, sight, and hearing and other senses that are contextualized by active practices, as well as both symbolic and pre-linguistic means of sense-making. Sense and sense-making are

> closely related and often implied by each other. The sense[s are] both a reaching out to the world as a source of information and an understanding of that world so gathered. This sensuous experience and understanding is grounded in previous experience and expectation, each dependent on sensual and sensory capacities and educational training and cultural conditioning.
>
> (Rodaway 1994:5)

The senses emerge through a process of objectification of one's sensations. In short, somatic experience is mediated by reflexivity—at both symbolic and alinguistic levels; carnal sensations "become objects to ourselves" (Mead 1938: 429). Flesh and organs bestow the capacity to sense, but those are merely the raw materials by which we fashion somatic experience. As the Huxley example shows, the senses are subject to and constituents of a system of somatic interaction that are situated in both cultural worlds (structured by "somatic rules") and existential worlds (comprised of sensorial transformation, multimodality, and emergence). Between the cultural and existential, human sensory experience is contingent on or mediated by *somatic work.*

Inspired by such popular sociological concepts as identity work (Snow and Anderson 1987) and emotional labor (Hochschild 1983), we offer the following definition: somatic work refers to the range of linguistic and alinguistic reflexive experiences and activities by which individuals interpret create, extinguish, maintain, interrupt, and/or communicate somatic sensations that are congruent with personal, interpersonal, and/or cultural notions of moral, aesthetic, and/or logical desirability.

We perform somatic work according to negotiated "somatic rules" that vary by personal, interpersonal, contextual, social, cultural, material, geographic, and historical circumstances. These circumstances are as symbolic as corporeal, as cultural as physical, as ritualized as creatively improvised. In short, we manage carnal sensations by performing somatic work according to negotiated somatic rules.

Somatic work is a more or less original moniker. Its origin lies deep in the history of interactionist and classic pragmatist thought, and several scholars associated with these traditions have closely approximated what we imply with the concept of somatic work. For example, in his study of marijuana users, Howard Becker (1963) suggests that the "taste" required for perceiving and interpreting the effects of marijuana is mediated by reflexive processes. Sensing is a social practice, rather than purely a chemical or physiological effect. Thus, marijuana users must perform reflexive work to cultivate a multiperspectival sense of appreciation for otherwise "vague impulses and desires" about the kind of sensory experience it affords, how that experience may be interpreted, and what it means (Becker 1963:42). Just as the sensory experience of marijuana use "is a function of the individual's conception of marijuana and of the uses to which it can be put" (Becker 1963:42), so is any other sensory experience. Sensory experience hinges on somatic work that is reflexive, pragmatic, phenomenological, and emergent from dialectic body skills (Ingold 2000) where meanings emerge at the intersection of the perceiver's sensory biography and existing social habits of uses of the senses (see Dewey 2002; Simmel 1997).

Becker was not the first to remark on the intentionality of sensory perception. Merleau-Ponty (1962) and Dewey (1929, 1934, 2002) also highlighted the active meaning-making potential of human senses. For Dewey, in particular, "habit" constitutes the epitome of his general theory of organic interaction "between elements of human nature and the environment, natural and social" (Dewey 2002:10). As he put it (2002:14), "habits are acquired" functions which manifest skills of sensory and motor organs, cunning or craft, and objective materials. They assimilate objective energies, and eventuate in command of environment. They require order, discipline, and manifest technique. They have a beginning, middle, and end (Dewey 2002:15). Habits are not synonymous with senses, yet for Dewey (2002:32) "habitual attitudes . . . govern concrete sensory materials." We suggest that somatic work is a processual by-product of the constitution of habit as a working mechanism that "filters all the material that reaches our perception and thought" and "adds new qualities and rearranges what is received" (Dewey 2002:32).

Somatic work is a useful concept for explaining how complex meaning can originate in the senses, even in the absence of abstract symbols. Meanings can be "had" and "known," according to Dewey. As Rochberg-Halton (1982) has pointed out, we experience meanings first by virtue of their *qualitative immediacy*. We sense certain objects for their immediate qualities and our carnal affective knowledge does not depend on abstract associations—such as the associations necessary to connect words with their referents. Humans *can* know, sense, and thus craft meaning carnally, without the necessary aid of abstract symbols. We then filter these sensory qualities by deploying the qualifying practices of somatic work.

Mead also contributes to our understanding of somatic work by suggesting that it is through such senses as "vision and touch [that] we build up a physical world" (McCarthy 1984:107). "Kinesthetic sensation" (Mead 1938:428, 429)—touching, feeling, grasping, holding, and relinquishing objects of our environment—constitutes "physical things which are in a real sense the products of [our] own hands" (Mead 1934:249). As Mitchell (2002:83, 97) suggests, kinesthetic sensation (a specific form of somatic work) is a type of bricolage: "we touch and turn and weigh in hand, and from these textured resistances, derive senses of our own physical scope and attributes." However, while Mitchell (2002:97) was interested in how "bricolage, utilitarian eroticism, extends self-discovery into the material realm" we are interested in Mead's original formulation: how somatic work, as a carnal form of bricolage, implicates self-discovery at the intersection of the corporeal and symbolic. The bricolage of somatic work "calls forth the whole of the corporeal self" (Mitchell 2002:83) and in a distinctively reflexive manner by which somatic experiences "become a physical object over and against the physical thing" (Mead 1938:428).

Thus we arrive at an interactionist "root image" (Blumer 1969) for a sociology of somatic experience. Vision is not necessarily sight; to listen is not necessarily to hear; to touch (or feel) implicates more than nerve endings; and so forth. Somatic experience is fundamentally reflexive: carnal sensations "become objects to ourselves" (Mead 1938:429), in both linguistic and pre-linguistic forms of meaning-making, which we actively manage through forms of somatic work and in the context of negotiated somatic rules. In sum, somatic work serves as both a unifying concept and as a subject matter—a concept and a subject matter upon which we will expand in later chapters.

***

In light of all we have suggested thus far, the organization of our book follows a simultaneously pedagogical and analytical plan. The book is comprised of two parts, with a total of eight chapters. Within each part, each chapter is structured around a broad field of social and cultural concern. Part I ("Understanding Sensory Studies") builds the conceptual edifice of our work—all the framing and roofing, as it were, that frames our approach to the senses. Following this introductory chapter, Chapter 2 is about the body, and about how bodily dynamics—such as health, healing, illness, movement, gender, habit, the emotions, and sexuality—intersect with the senses. Chapter 3 focuses on performance, and thus on the performativity of sensing. As interactionists, our approach to the senses relies heavily on notions of action, hence this chapter illustrates how the sociality of sensing interplays with ritualization, drama, play, ceremony, art, and spectacle. Chapter 4 is about sensuous scholarship. With a focus on ethnography and qualitative research that entails embodied interaction between people and researchers, we detail how research can be made sensuous, and provide a rationale for why it should be so.

If the first part of the book is the basic frame of our house, Part II ("Doing Sensory Research") contains all the furniture and interior decorations that make our building truly our own. In this part, we concentrate less on laying out basic historical, substantive, and broad theoretical and methodological foundations. Instead, we engage more deeply with original empirical material and aim to deepen the reach of our research in key directions. Chapter 5 focuses on self and identity, and on how the senses and sensations constitute uniquely somatic dimensions of subjectivity. Chapter 6 is about place and time, and therefore about how our sensing grounds our existence in biography, individual and collective memory, history, and place. Chapter 7 concentrates on order, control, and deviance. Here, we examine somatic rules and alignment, power, and the sociality of sensing. Chapter 8 is about communication, and in particular about the roles that the senses and sensations play in media and popular culture, as well as in consumer culture and material culture. Driven by our data and personal experiences, these chapters stand out as diverse ways in which sensory research can be conducted.

By organizing our book's chapters in this manner, we hope to show both students and scholars with an interest in fields cognate to the social study of senses—for example, the sociology or anthropology of the body—that combining theoretical elements, empirical traditions, and concepts across fields enhances both the study of the senses and whatever other fields they may be interested in (e.g. the study of the body). Also, by including within each chapter literature review, research data, and theory, we hope to advance conceptual frameworks while shedding light on interesting human practices in both an analytical and a narrative fashion. Finally, throughout the book, insofar as our genre of writing allows, we hope to speak *about* the senses as much as *through* and *for* the senses.

2

THE SENSUAL BODY

"I discovered the sensations of my clitoris long before I ever properly identified the organ, the source of all the magic," writes Jessica, a twenty-one-year-old student at Minnesota State University:

> I was probably about nine or ten. I had been playing around with myself—not really masturbating, just spelunking my "down there"—and I pulled back some flesh and discovered this amazingly sensitive little knob (it almost felt a little dangerous). It was this hidden, private thing that I gazed at with some hesitancy. My first thought was something along the lines of "What the hell is *that*?!"

Like Jessica, many women rarely acquire formal, or even informal, written or verbal information about the clitoris until their mid- to late teens. Because formal sexual education in North America (at least) is inadequate, because parents are often embarrassed to talk about such things, and because popular discourses generally hide the clitoris under the hood of secrecy, most women come to know the clitoris first through their own touch. That is, in this case, *sensual information typically comes before conceptual information*; touch provides most women with knowledge that parents, formal education, peers, the media, and other agents of socialization do not and/or cannot explore in the same way. But touch is not a transparent medium. Many women discover their clitoris long before they become fully acquainted with the pleasing sensations that different touch techniques provide. This carnal awareness of one's own body continues to develop and change over time, over repeated touching—and that is precisely the subject of Dennis, Phillip, and Desiree Wiesen's (2007) study of women's recollections of the discovery of their clitoris, from which these data come. Indeed, as Jill (age twenty) writes,

> I discovered my clitoris when I was in third grade. So I was probably about eight. I didn't really know what was going on. I just knew that when I touched a certain spot it would feel really different than when I would touch other places. This discovery usually came along when I couldn't sleep at night.

Studying women's discovery of the clitoris to understand gender and sexual dynamics of touch and sensuous meaning-making, we learned that women often spoke of their touching experiences in similar ways: clitoral sensations are usually something they discover entirely for themselves in confidential, clandestine somatic explorations that provided a measure of privacy, easy sexual access to the genitals, and perhaps motivation to search for more intense pleasure as well. Ann's (age twenty-one) testimonial is a good example: "I remember discovering my clit when I was fairly young—I was around six or seven years old. Lying in my bed trying to go to sleep, I remember putting my hand down there and feeling around. I discovered I liked how it felt to touch it." Although unaware that "it" had a name, by discovering its pleasing sensations, Ann and many other women defined their clitoris as valuable and meaningful because it felt good. It is as if they did not quite know what it was, but they felt, carnally, that it "had" meaning (Dewey 2002). How is this possible?

In this chapter we more fully unpack these dynamics. Namely, we discuss how *the body makes sense*: how the body perceives, how it understands, how it knows, and how that is made possible because of sensual experience. We often think of knowledge as an exclusively mental affair. For example, we read a book and we acquire information, or we listen to a lecture and we learn something new. To be sure, those activities of the "mind" (Crossley 2006) are common ways of knowing, but cognition and verbal information are not the only sources of knowledge. The human body—through its senses and sensations—is also a source and object of knowledge. Therefore, on the one hand, it might be useful to think of sensations as comprising a language of their own. Indeed, we might argue that the

> senses comprise our first language. Long before we acquire the capacity to code, comprehend, and communicate in symbolic and linguistic forms, we have already mastered the intimate idioms of sight, sound, touch, taste, and smell. We retain and refine that somatic fluency and, for the rest of our lives, sensations are necessarily "both a reaching out to the world and a *source of information* and *an understanding* of that world so gathered" (Rodaway 1994:5, emphasis added)—a principal means by which we may know and understand. One might further argue that this partially accounts

> for the powerful, emotional and evocative nature of sensory experience and knowledge and the intellectual understandings that are made possible because of them.
>
> (Waskul 2009:655–656)

On the other hand, although the metaphor of "senses as language" might be useful, we have to be careful. Language is symbolic and sensations can only be *made symbolic* and only to a limited extent. What is unique about bodily ways of knowing is that, unlike the mind, they neither necessitate language nor are easily articulated through language. The body has different ways of "understanding," of finding and creating meaning. The body *makes sense* because, in part, the body *is sense* (Vannini and Waskul 2006). While "it" may lack symbolic meaning—whether "it" is an unnamed piece of flesh that turns out later to be called a clitoris or something else—"it" is bountiful with other forms of meaning that did not need to be "uncovered" or "constructed" because we carnally inhabit them at all times (see Ingold 2000). As we will soon detail, these ways of knowing are sourced from iconic meanings (Peirce 1931) that are rich with what Dewey (2002) called "qualitative immediacy."

Ways of knowing through (and about) our body are multiple, irregular, and often complex. For example, bodily awareness may be hidden or disappear from consciousness until a "sensory intensification" (Leder 1990:71), such as a feeling of ill-being or pleasure, unfolds, allowing body parts "waiting like tools in a box to be used by conscious resolve" (Dewey 2002:25; also see Leder 1990). This is precisely what Kari (age twenty), one of our study's participants, reports: "I guess I could say I was little, like ten or eleven, when I discovered the good feeling of it being rubbed . . . *I knew what 'it' was before I knew it was a clitoris*" (emphasis added). Experiences like Kari's cannot be understood through language alone; the body is a prime site of alinguistic knowledge (Dewey 1934, 2002). As Frank (1995:27) suggests, "The body is not mute, but it is inarticulate; it does not use speech but it begets it." This form of linguistically "pre-reflexive experience" (Csordas 1990:6) is fully embodied, and is the basis of many manifestations of sensual embodiment. Under the broad umbrella of the "sensual body"—which could address innumerable topics—we will focus our attention on four of these manifestations of sensual embodiment: movement, health and illness, gender, and sexual embodiment. We now turn to these and conclude by returning to our study of sensations of the clitoris.

MOVEMENT

Natural scientists identify two senses connected to the experience and practice of movement: the *vestibular sense* and the *kinesthetic sense*. The vestibular sense allows us to perceive direction, acceleration, and movement in space. This sense has another function: to perceive and achieve balance—a function that some other scholars attribute to another sense, called *equilibrioception*. On the other hand, the kinesthetic sense—also known as *proprioception*—allows us to perceive the relative position and movement of different parts of the body. Juggling, for example, among innumerable other activities, requires keen cultivation of proprioception. Together, the vestibular and the kinesthetic senses are responsible for almost all of human action, if we take into account the fact that, almost inevitably, most forms of practical engagement of the world by human beings require bodily movement and (re)positioning in space. From walking to grabbing, from scratching to jumping, from standing to all forms of embodied self-expression, the moving body is able to strive for survival, connect with others, avoid danger, and manipulate the environment. Ingold (2000:166) captures the importance of movement nicely when he writes: "locomotion not cognition must be the starting point for the study of perceptual activity."

Recently, a handful of scholars has begun to study movement as sensual experience by examining the sensations experienced in sports. One of the key exponents of this movement, Andrew Sparkes (2009), has reviewed this growing body of literature and found it to be an important corrective to perspectives that examine the moving sporting body as nothing but a signifying vehicle of cultural codes. Similarly, Hockey and Collinson (2007:116) argue that better understanding of sport "demands engaging with the phenomenology of the body, particularly the sensuous and sensing sporting body."

Obviously, we agree with these scholars. Moving the body is also an important manifestation of what we call somatic work. To move and seek equilibrium is a deeply social activity. Think, for example, of how rhythm is so regulated in sports (e.g. there are only a few seconds to shoot a basketball or spike a football; see Hockey and Collinson 2007), or how aesthetic conventions stipulate the quality of balance in such sports as ski-jumping, gymnastics, figure-skating, and synchronized swimming. People constantly move to achieve sensations that feel "just right," and that feeling is deeply shaped by socialization to what is socially desirable. Consider dance, for example. As Potter (2008:449) describes through her ethnography of dancers, they struggle mightily to understand aesthetic conventions and achieve good form "as they walk, balance, spin, stretch, crouch, jump, curve, fall, bend, toss the limbs into space, run, shake, remain still, crawl, roll, or lift someone during daily training."

In her study of ballet dancers, Kleiner (2009) explores how, through highly self-conscious interactions with self and others, the dancers learn how it feels to embody what an audience sees; and, in the process of training their bodies, how they strive to achieve an institutionalized aesthetic. This embodiment of technique facilitates a reflexive experience while performing that both evokes and suppresses the mind in a studied and trained sensual absorption in movement and music. Kleiner (2009:248) explains:

Embodiment of ballet technique requires a long-term project of comparing each movement to an ideal, and slowly training the body to approach the proper form. It involves encountering a dual self-consciousness, both of movements that are continually adjusted in a highly disciplining environment and of bodily forms that are not controllable by movement. Dancers encounter and battle this self-consciousness by adjusting the appearance of the body to approach the shape of static requirements such as weight, refining movements to bring them closer to proper technique, or leaving the training context. They also self-consciously ingrain specific choreography during rehearsals, with the goal of not having to think during the performance. By self-consciously training and adjusting their bodies, dancers prepare themselves to avoid activating the "reflective self" (self-consciousness) during performance, thereby facilitating flow.

Of course, in the context of sporting activity, body movements cannot be easily confined to one sensorial dimension alone. Sport is a dance of synaesthetic moves, of deliberate resolutions. "The angle of the head and torso, for example, or stride length, arm movement, and leg cadence," write Hockey and Collinson (2007:119), "are all particular corporeal choices." We make these choices on the basis of sensations like nociception (the sense of pain), touch, the aural and visual dimensions of movement, and so forth. Consider, for example, how cricket players choose their bats. As Sparkes (2009:22) describes: "Each [bat] is picked up, held out at arm's length, swung, twisted and swished through the air" in imagination and anticipation of the flight of the ball toward the sweet spot of the bat. Somatic work is also performed when seeking to perfect movement after someone has undergone an injury and as she attempts to re-educate her body to simple skills, such as running. As Hockey (2006:188) reports in an entry from the daily diary he kept on the multi-sensorial experience of running and pain:

> [We] initially tried some tiny 10-meter trots with rests in between, but to our consternation [we] are like babies! Like drunks we stagger all over the place. No coordination, legs out of kilter with arms, unused to the effort so breathing is ragged, legs do not seem to fit with the torso, and head feels wobbly and heavy. Even these baby trots empty us, compounding the problem.

Circumstances in which an individual needs to train or retrain himself to ordinary sensory habits—such as re-learning how to walk or run after an accident—can teach us much about embodiment as a socialization process. Learning to breathe according to the standards practiced by yoga teachers, for example, highlights the degree to which sensations of rhythm, balance, and movement are the outcomes of active, reflexive efforts (both linguistically and non-linguistically). Or take the socialization of walking: different cultures and subcultures (and different gendered bodies) teach their members that certain ways of walking (e.g. with your chest out, looking confident and proud, striding along a fashion runway, or swaying like a gangster) evoke desirable sensations, and others evoke undesirable ones (see Edensor 2000; Ingold and Vergunst 2008; Urry 2000, 2007).

Indeed, walking is not as natural as we believe it to be. To move appropriately is to display not only motor skills but also social skills. For instance, throughout her fieldwork among the Anlo-Ewe in southeastern Ghana, Kathryn Geurts (2003) repeatedly heard about the sense the locals called *azolizozo*. This is the kinesthetic sense involved in all forms of movement, including walking. But in Anlo-Ewe culture, *azolizozo* is deeply intertwined with another sense (albeit something that is not necessarily referred to as a sense in the West): morality. Morality is an association of kinesthetic qualities and sensations, and of sensible dispositions or moral character (*azolime*). *Azolizozo* and *azolime* share the root *zo*: to move. In a particularly evocative passage, Geurts (2003:188–189) writes:

> Aaron and Kobla never seemed to go straight to the well when their mother sent them to fetch water. I often observed them "horsing around" as they made their way through the compound and out the gate to the community well in the village where we lived. One day, as I watched them running in circles, chasing each other, walking backwards, and swinging their buckets to and fro, I heard their mother shouting in a distressed voice something about how they were walking *lugulugu*. My ears perked up when I heard that adverb, *lugulugu*, as I had recently begun making a list of different kinds of walks or styles of comportment. I already knew that one could *zo kadzakadza* (walk like a lion), or *zo minyaminya* (walk stealthily, as if eavesdropping), or *zo megbemegbe* (walk backwards, leaving deceptive footprints). As Kobla's mother shouted at them from behind her kitchen wall, I watched them darting from one side of the compound to the other, swaying perilously on the outer edge of a foot, feigning to nearly fall down, and evidently imitating their mother's charge that they were moving *lugulugu* on their way to the well . . . I began by asking Elaine, my research assistant, what *lugulugu* really meant. She explained that while a word such as *zo lugulugu* referred in the first instance to bodily motions such as swaying, tarrying, dawdling, or moving as if drunk, it could also be used to refer to a person's character. In response to a daughter's statement that "Kofi is the man I want to marry," Elaine explained that parents might discourage the young woman with the retort, "*Tsyo! Ame lugulugu*!" The expression reveals the parents' perception that Kofi was a *lugulugu* man: a person who did not simply move in a tarrying or dawdling fashion, but a person who was not serious—an aimless, irresponsible fellow.

HEALTH, ILLNESS, AND DEATH

Like movement, health and illness are sensations. We are able to experience these bodily conditions through the sense called *nociception*. This works in conjunction with touch when we experience pain through cutaneous exposure and it works with other interoceptive neurological systems when experiences of pain are visceral or joint- and bone-related. Despite the fact that nociception has never made it into the "top five" best-known senses, its importance is undeniable because, of all the senses, it is the most clearly connected to dynamics of survival. (Closely related to nociception is the sense of *thermoception*, which allows us to sense temperature both within and outside of our bodies.)

As said, health and illness are sensations, but we often think of them as states of being. This is arguably because sensations of health and illness are tightly organized around a body of knowledge that allows all of us to *translate* subjective bodily sensations into objective states of being (diagnoses) that can be verified, measured, and controlled for medical purposes. Take, for instance, how we, as parents, may react to the morning whining of a schoolchild:

"Daddy, I don't feel good."

"You sounded fine to me a few minutes ago when you were playing in your bedroom."

"But I feel kind of sick."

"Well, you don't look sick to me. I think you're just faking it because you don't want to go to school."

"No!"

"Well, let me check your temperature . . . See? You're not warm at all. You're going to school. Period!"

Parents are not being heartless in such circumstances. Rather, as an interoceptive sense, nociception is subject to the scrutiny of *other* senses (and the sense-making practices of others' senses), which allows for the objectification (and validation) of experiences of pain. This scrutiny allows for private sensation to be made public and for sensations derived through the working of one sense to be translated through the working of other (and others') senses. Thus, from a deeply private sensation, pain undergoes a great degree of *semiotic and somatic translation* to acquire a social life. This process of semiotic and somatic translation is a form of somatic work.

Pangs of pain are carnal sensations that "awaken" the body into awareness of itself (Leder 1990). As we first perceive these noxious sensations—in the immediate moments when perception begins to unfold—we cannot easily define their nature through words. These are moments marked by raw feeling: sensing unmediated by words or even by emotions. These textures of pain—though the same can be said for sensations yielded by all senses under the same circumstances—can be said to have a qualitative immediacy (Dewey 2002) that only a sense can know and comprehend in its purity. During this primordial state—which can be very fleeting—things are as they are: unique in and of themselves. Or perhaps they are what they are by virtue of the fact that they closely *resemble* similar experiences of the same or a nearly related kind. Following Peirce (1931) we can call these sensations *iconic*.

Humans are social beings, and it does not take long before private, iconic sensations become subject to a scrutiny that allows us to share them with others. As our attention narrows on a noxious or pleasant sensation, we may feel various emotions. And we may begin to search for words to describe such a sensation, and perhaps relate its nature to other people. For example, medical experts use our description to begin to look for a host of different signs (called symptoms) to produce a diagnosis and make sense of our experience. The signs they seek out are of the iconic type, but also of the *indexical* type. Whereas making sense of noxious feelings in an iconic way allows physicians to establish—through relations of token-type resemblance—what something may or may not be (e.g. "It sounds like pneumonia, therefore it must be pneumonia and not a common cough"), making sense of noxious feelings indexically allows them to conclude that the somatic sign is the effect of a predetermining cause. This form of interpretive work is, for example, the basis of auscultation (Rice 2003; Sterne 2001): through the use of a stethoscope, a physician may infer that a wheezing sound in the lungs is caused by the presence of a particular virus.

A third type of interpretive somatic work occurs at the *symbolic* level, where we do not experience and understand sensations for what they are or resemble, or for what they indicate, but for what they represent or refer to. We may attribute ill sensations to having engaged in untoward conduct or being a victim of a witch's malicious spell (Stroeken 2008) or because we have lost our dignity and independence (Waskul and Van der Riet 2002). In such cases it is thus perfectly commonsensical that the performance of healing be aided by rituals invested with special symbolic properties (Laderman and Roseman 1996; Roseman 1993).

Symbolic, indexical, and iconic interpretive work allows us to make sense of a sensation, to know what it is, what caused it, and what it stands for. Performing these kinds of somatic work, we come to know our body in multiple, nuanced, and at times even contradictory ways. As with any form of hermeneutic work, such somatic work always takes place in contexts that are shaped by numerous characteristics. One of the most important characteristics that we wish to examine in this chapter is an individual's past, and in particular what is known as a sensory biography (Desjarlais 2003; Seremetakis 1994) or somatic career (Waskul, Vannini, and Wilson 2009). Sensory biographies and somatic careers (more fully explored later) are, of course, not just individual affairs. Every biography is woven within a precise historical context.

For example, Robert Desjarlais's (2003) interpretive biography of Ghang Lama is very attentive to how age, historical context, and individual activities shape personal patterns of making sense of illness and death. Desjarlais focuses in particular on dynamics of vision, which he finds to be particularly important in Nepal Yolmo's Buddhist culture. Vision gives form to personal life and the world as a whole. Vision is equated to presence, to the visibility and meaningfulness of one's actions. Desjarlais (2003:160) finds that as Mheme—or Ghang Lama—ages, he begins to lose his presence and visibility in this world: "Memories, dreams, his appetite, his body, his physical strength and abilities, the faces of friends, the confidence of others, the times of his youth—all these had disappeared like words written on water." Mheme's carnal experiences of illness and death are therefore best understood when situated within the sensory order of Yolmo society and history and his own sensory biography—which provides him with the resources to make sense of his body's sensations.

GENDER

Many claim that men and women do things, and experience them, differently. Investigations on how men and women sense differently are no exception. Thus, Classen (1997), for example, has shown that throughout different historical periods men and women have been believed to perceive things differently and have therefore been subject to normative prescriptions and expectations that may have contributed to developing those very differences. Through Synnott's (1993) valuable historical investigation, we also learn that men and women, among other differences, reputedly:

- communicate differently through touch, and perceive touching sensations differently, often resulting in conflicting sexual needs;
- rely on sight differentially, with men being supposedly more visual than women and women often suffering from men's sexualizing and objectifying gaze;
- are socialized differently, as little girls are touched more often and looked at more intensely;
- are believed and expected to smell differently, and to enjoy different fragrances.

Even though most authors are aware that their sweeping generalizations have limits and that there is as much variation within gender groups as across genders, such claims are often imbued with a great degree of commonsense knowledge and thus credibility, and in turn readers cannot help but come away with the feeling that gender differences—whether by nature or nurture—are matters of fact.

Of course, the senses have been invested with gender values throughout history. Anthropologist and historian Constance Classen finds that in spite of the commonly held belief—originated during the Enlightenment—that the senses are neutral media, historical evidence dating back to pre-modernity shows that the senses have traditionally been infused with binary gender ideologies. For example, it has been believed that women's body temperature is colder than men's, and that women have a more acute fragrance than men—a fragrance that is cunningly used to seduce men. As Classen (1997:4–5) explains, sensory hierarchies are strong and pervasive:

> Along with being assigned different sensory qualities, men and women were associated with different sensory processes. At the most fundamental level, men were associated with the mind and soul and women with the body and senses . . . While the senses were feminine when opposed to male rationality, however, *within* the domain of the senses, gender distinctions applied as well. In the case of each sense, men would typically be associated with what were thought to be the nobler qualities of that sense, and women with the more ignoble. As regards sight, for example, men were ideally imagined to employ this sense for intellectual activities such as studying and devising plans, while women made use of it for the sensual ends of acquiring gaudy clothes and looking at themselves in the mirror. Men were deemed to use the sense of hearing, similarly, to listen to weighty discourses and lectures, while women employed their hearing to attend to frivolous gossip and love talk. While each sense was considered to have superior and inferior uses, the senses of sight and hearing were held to be more closely associated with the "higher" functions of the mind, and the other senses with the "lower" functions of the body. In accordance with the mind/body, male/female duality outlined above, men tended to be linked with the "rational" senses of sight and hearing, and women with the "corporeal" senses of smell, taste and touch. The social consequences of this gendering of the senses were multifold. The fact that the "male" senses of sight and hearing were classified as "distance" senses, and the "female" senses of smell, taste and touch were characterized as "proximity" senses, was interpreted to mean that men were suited for "distance activities," such as travelling and governing, while women were made to stay at home. Furthermore, the customary association of sight and hearing with mental functions, and of smell, taste and touch with bodily functions, made intellectual endeavors such as the arts and sciences the prerogative of men, while women were in charge of caring for the bodily needs of their families.

Viewing the senses as yet another domain of the alleged schism that separates the genders, however, can yield only partial insight. It might be more useful instead—or, if anything, more interesting—to reflect on precisely *how the gendering of the senses occurs*: through what precise processes and dynamics (Classen 1997). For example, women and men *are perceived* differently and those differential perceptions are primarily visual. As Stone (1962) has described, we routinely assign a social identity to people on the basis of the visual cues their bodies display. Clothes, hair, and makeup play a key role in this visual process, and we often classify people's bodies into gender categories by relying exclusively on this sensory process. An interesting example of this is suggested by what Kessler and McKenna (1978) call the gender attribution process. They write about a child who, upon seeing a photograph of someone in a business suit, contends that the photographed person is "a man, because he has a pee-pee" (Kessler and McKenna 1978:154). Obviously, the child cannot see a penis in the photo, but he imputes it to the person on the basis of visual signs of known masculinity (the business attire). What this case illustrates is that gender is thus imputed, or attributed, to others on the basis of the surfaces (appearance, conduct, etc.) that are detectable in social interaction.

An extensive body of research on visual appearance suggests that men's and women's bodies *are made to look* different across cultures, and these visual performances of gender would strike anyone as more significant than the anatomical basis they are supposed to signify or accentuate. For example, hair and dress are styled differently by men and women (Akou 2007; Synnott 1993), different ways of dressing are key tools in the presentation of self (Goffman 1959, 1974, 1979), children's bodies are adorned differently during rites of passage marking their bodily growth (e.g. circumcision, first menstruation), ornaments such as lip and ear discs and penis sheaths are used to emphasize body shapes (O'Hanlon 1989; Seeger 1975), and social norms and expectations regarding tanning vary across gender (Vannini and McCright 2004). Among Greek villagers, Welters (1995) finds that men's and women's clothes even sound different, as the women's jewelry, made of coins and worn as part of their traditional dress, makes rather loud clicking noises when they move. These different performances of the gendered body illustrate that social scripts lay out clear gendered sensory roles and cast social actors into them, allowing for differential sensory socialization patterns.

In light of such different socialization patterns, it is not uncommon for most men and women to learn to sense the world differently. Later in this chapter, we will return to our examination of how women come to discover and learn about their clitoris, and how they experience their sexual bodies through masturbation. While it is rather normal, and even expected, for young boys to discuss "woodies" and sexual curiosities openly with one another (e.g. Fine 1987), different somatic rules pertinent to sexuality—as well as for other sensual experiences—exist for girls. We develop this argument in the next section.

SEXUAL EMBODIMENT

The phrase "carnal knowledge" means "to know by the flesh." While legally and colloquially the phrase has only meant sexual knowledge—and intercourse in particular—"to know by the flesh" is the binding theme of this entire chapter. Still, like movement, health, and illness, carnal sexual knowledge is another significant if not universal form of sensual embodiment with unique characteristics of its own. Indeed, like eating and drinking, sex might be among the greatest expressions of sensuality. Moreover, sexual embodiment is a paradigmatic case of sensual embodiment—somatic work is the means by which the person and body know and cultivate sexual arousal through carnal sensual experience.

While it is probable that sexual desire is influenced by hormones, that is not the end but the beginning of the story. Indeed, "sexuality can be thought of as an institution defined by shared meaning" (Rye and Meaney 2007:29) and sexual arousal entails what Davis (1983) often referred to as a "sensual slide" into "erotic reality." "Whoever moves from everyday to erotic reality," Davis wrote (1983:13; emphasis in original), "experiences a *lascivious shift* in relevances in the temporal, spatial, social, and physical dimensions along which he [or she] organizes his [or her] world—a sexual effect analogous to the Doppler effect in physics." Furthermore, that increasing intensity of sexual arousal changes the way people perceive and experience the body and its sensations, themselves, and each other. As Davis (1983:33–34) notes,

> first, it seems to intensify their experience of physical characteristics relative to social and psychological ones . . . Second, the sexually aroused experience the body as more sharply segregated from its circumstances than do the sexually unaroused. In short, the self, abstract and dispersed in everyday reality, becomes embodied and localized in erotic reality.

Sexual pleasure, like pain, has the power to embody the self fully in the exceedingly narrow spatial and temporal zone of the here and now, either alone or among immediate lovers, which partly accounts for why people often describe the experience of sexual arousal as "distracting" while, in truth, it is a highly *focused* state of sensual embodiment(s).

Sexual desire and arousal are not one and the same thing. On the one hand, "physiological-genital sexual arousal may occur without conscious awareness" (Regan and Berscheid 1999:16). For example, it seems that not all women are able to report their level of physical genital sexual arousal (Heiman 1975), and a male erection is not necessarily indicative of sexual desire. After all, some men playfully refer to a NRB ("no reason boner"). In fact, even the occurrence of sexual activity does not necessarily imply desire: one study found that over 50 percent of undergraduate women and almost 25 percent of men engaged in non-coercive but undesired sexual activities (Regan 1997). Indeed, people have sex for a wide variety of motives that may be unrelated to their own sexual desire—such as indulging your lover's desire for a "birthday bang." Meanwhile, lack of sexual activity is certainly no reliable sign of disinterest.

In short, sexual embodiment requires carnal reflexivity—a sensuous awareness that one is aroused—what some have called "subjective sexual arousal" (Mosher, Barton-Henry, and Green 1988). As William James (1983:486) put it, "We desire to feel, to have, to do all sorts of things which at the moment are not felt, had, or done," and subjective sexual arousal "is the awareness that one is *now* experiencing certain physiological and/or genital reactions" (Regan and Berscheid 1999:17; emphasis in original). For these reasons, understanding sexual embodiment as a passive state of being—something merely triggered by external stimuli (a sexy body, romantic settings, or even the touch of someone else) or internal biochemical states (androgens, testosterone, etc.)—is woefully inadequate. Sexual embodiment is an active state of being that hinges on reflexive somatic work, and this is precisely what is missing in purely mechanical formulations of sexual arousal, such as Masters and Johnson's (1966) Human Sexual Response Cycle.

Sexual arousal is a highly specific "somatic mode of attention" (Csordas 1993) whereby people direct attention *to* bodily sensation and are paying attention *with* their body, whether alone or in the embodied presence of others. This is why the gynecological exam is rarely, if ever, defined as "sexual" (or pleasing), even though it contains most of the basic elements of erotic interaction—two people, nudity, the spreading of legs, the touching of breasts, and penetration of the vagina (Henslin and Biggs 1971). It may also explain why most men do not conclude their prostate exams by asking the doctor, "Was it good for you?" Indeed, "although our bodies are always present, we do not always attend to and with them" (Csordas 1993:139). Attending to the body requires somatic work.

In sexual arousal, we pay attention to and with our bodily sensations, and often in scripted actions and interactions (Gagnon and Simon 1973) that we *define* as carnal sexual sensations—touches, tastes, smells, sounds, movements—and experience as pleasurable. In fact, some theorists argue that sex *is* pleasure (see Abramson and Pinkerton 1995). However, pleasure is not only in the eye of the beholder but socially scripted, culturally defined, reinforced, and regulated—as we illustrate in our next section.

SENSUAL WAYS OF KNOWING

Touch and the Discovery of Qualitative Immediacy

Like most sensations, touch often recedes to the back of consciousness. Take, for example, the clothes you are wearing right now. Their presence is subtle, but it is there if you pay attention. As you read these words, perhaps you may even become more aware of how they feel: how your shoes feel on your feet, whether they fit tight and make you a bit uncomfortable, or whether they feel just right. Perhaps you may begin to reflect on the objects around you that "touch you." How comfortable is the seat you are sitting on? Is it cushioned enough or too hard on your buttocks or back? Indeed, most of the time, these sensations require little "minding"—that is, little cognitive reflection. But at other times, in rarer circumstances, our body senses qualities that we are not so easily capable of reflecting on. These rarer circumstances can teach us a lot about "somatic modes of attention" (Csordas 1993). In our study of how women come to discover their clitoris for the first time (Waskul, Vannini, and Wiesen 2007), we found that women most often discover this sexual organ when they possess little or no information about it. This circumstance enables a unique experience that is marked by the presence of intensely meaningful sensations and by the absence of meaningful cognitive information. We refer to this absence of information as "symbolic clitoridectomy."

By "symbolic clitoridectomy" (see Ogletree and Ginsburg 2000; see also Bennett 1993 on "critical" clitoridectomy), we refer to the silence, the taboo, and the failure to identify or define the clitoris. Symbolic clitoridectomy is a bracketing of the clitoris by means of linguistic and discursive erasure. It most often requires women to confront and negotiate what we call "symbolic purgatory": a situation in which women discover a sensation long before they fully acquire the symbolic knowledge (i.e. cognitive information) with which to make sense of it. All of the women who participated in our study reported a significant gap between the carnal discovery of the iconic sensations generated by touching their clitoris and full acquisition of the symbolic knowledge that the clitoris is a standard part of female genitalia. This purgatory period begs provocative questions about meaning, language, somatic experience, and, in this case, their interstices in what is generally deemed the most private realm of the corporeal body.

As an *object*, the clitoris is an anatomical organ. But as a *subject*, it is contested social terrain: an epicenter of female sexuality in which pleasure and repression collide on an embodied fault line that is both private and public, political and existential, symbolic and corporeal. As an organ, the clitoris is a source of potentially pleasing sensuality, a sensuality that has an immediate quality to it. As an icon, not a symbol, the clitoris has multiple immediate meanings whose signification is negotiated in a variety of qualities, subjective sensations, experiences, and reflexive acts of sense-making. The great majority of studies that focus on how things come to mean what they do focus on linguistic meaning. Language and speech generally hinge on linguistic reflexivity: we interact with ourselves and others primarily through significant symbols. The same applies to the body: by use of symbols, we perceive, interact, and interpret our own body as much as we sense, interact with, and interpret the bodies of others. However, linguistic or symbolic reflexivity is limited (DeNora 1997; Rochberg-Halton 1982). Because the body is our "first property" (Simmel 1950:322n, 344), its "qualitative immediacy" (Dewey 1929, 1934) or firstness (Peirce 1931)—that is, the way it feels meaningful carnally—assures a ubiquitous source of sensation and iconic meaning. In other words, somatic experience is reflexive and meaningful even in the absence of significant symbols; and even in the relative absence of discourses, the qualitative immediacy of that experience is not culturally neutral.

How, exactly, do we experience the qualitative immediacy of corporeal sensations in the relative absence of symbolic meaning? Or, closer to our concerns here, what happens when we experience a part of our body when symbols for identification and meaning-making are relatively absent? In order to answer these questions, we asked a sample of university women to write in anonymous journals about how they recalled coming to find out about their clitoris. Their answers were brutally honest and incredibly revealing of both sensual and gender dynamics. Danielle (age twenty-one), for example, recalls her discovery as follows:

> The first time I remember having sensations, I was probably nine or ten years old, between fourth and fifth grade. I was climbing a pole on the playground and it felt good to climb upwards. I don't remember knowing or understanding what it meant at the time, just that it felt good. I remember not wanting anyone to know why I liked it, although I recall a girlfriend teasing me, so I figured she "knew" too. I don't recall too much from elementary and junior high [school] but I'm guessing I was about fourteen or fifteen when I was using a back massager and it fell into my lap. I suddenly realized what "that" feeling was. I knew I had a clit by then, but probably still had not been told that it was for pleasure. I put the massager away and tried to forget about what happened, but the next time I was home alone I decided to explore more. This is when I discovered that the vibrations felt the best on my clit. I liked it but I didn't want anyone to know.

As is apparent in Danielle's account, some women do not recall freely exploring their body as a child. Both Beth and Sara (both twenty years old) did not discover the pleasures of their clitoris until a book motivated carnal exploration. As Beth explains:

> I had begun reading more mature books that had sex in them, and it made me curious. So I started to experiment touching myself. I was in my bed at night and it was a new and thrilling experience . . . I believe I was in early junior high . . . I couldn't believe that my body could feel like that and that I had gone so long without knowing it existed.

Beth was surprised that she "had gone so long without knowing it existed," which is understandable considering that "the possibility of pleasure is literally in [her] own hands" (Plante 2006:144), and always had been.

According to our data, women generally discover the pleasures of the clitoris long before they know it has a name, a circumstance we described earlier as symbolic purgatory. Several women, such as Cheryl (age nineteen), remarked on this gap between somatic discovery and discursive knowledge:

> I didn't learn about the clitoris specifically until ninth grade (age fourteen). Before that I had learned about the female genitalia in a rather broad sense. I knew there was more to the female genitalia than just a vagina (learned from general discussion with my family/parents, not really any specific age), but I didn't know what each part was called. In ninth grade health class, my teacher passed out very detailed diagram pictures with everything labeled for both female and male genitalia . . . In the back of my mind, I vaguely connected the clitoris to the specific part that gave me the most pleasure.

Until learning that their "special spot" is a clitoris, some women—such as Sara—"just assumed that it was a part of the vagina but with no specific name." Other women, such as Ann (age twenty-one), "had no idea other people had a spot like this that felt good to touch." Somatic discovery is a sensual and carnal source of both meaning and information for the embodied self. However, it is not entirely language free. For example, our informants often use the euphemism "down there" to refer to the clitoris—with all its connotations of everything sexual, naughty, mysterious, unspeakable, devious, and so forth—and this clearly illustrates how even upon first encounter, the clitoris is neither confined to discursive darkness nor basking in symbolic transparency. The clitoris inhabits an intermediate state (purgatory), awaiting linguistic conceptualization, which is evident in Cheryl's recollection: "I knew for many years that it wasn't just a vagina *but [I] never really concerned myself with more than that*" (emphasis added). A similar waiting for discursive cues is equally apparent in the accounts of Jessica (age twenty-one; emphasis added) and Diana (age twenty-two; emphasis added): "I always knew there was more going on 'down there' than just a hole, but *until I was given names and info for the different parts I never really thought much about them*"; "I don't think I ever consciously thought about 'the thing down there' *until I learned it had a name.* Once it had a name it was something OK; something more real."

The *relative* muting of the clitoris is all the more significant because, as Rebecca (age twenty) claims, "it [the clitoris] does bring me great sexual pleasure, and when I think about it I usually think about the pleasure I get from it." More than mere vocabulary, language may well constitute a lexicon for experience; in this case, the experience of pleasure.

Generally, the women in our study were eventually relieved to learn "it" was a clitoris. Since language is a cultural stockpile of accepted meaning and truth, simply knowing "it" has a name validates and legitimizes the clitoris and a young woman's body, femininity, and sexuality. A word renders the clitoris a significant symbol—which is significant, indeed:

> I had spent months pleasuring myself before I learned what exactly I was using to do it. It was kind of nice to know my body was working properly.
>
> (Beth)

> I remember looking down there and kind of wondering about it, to find out later that it felt good, and then had a name. I think I was surprised that it had its own name. It was kind of nice to be able to label it though, and know that it was different from everything else down there. I was excited but embarrassed that I "knew."
>
> (Danielle)

Similarly, Ann writes, "It was a relief to finally know the name." However, as she also understandably adds, "I already knew it was normal, but I thought it was strange I had never learned its function." Her clitoris had been a part of her body all her life, she had already discovered its wonderful pleasures, and yet she was denied basic anatomical knowledge. More than just finding the whole experience "strange," some women were resentful: "As I became aware, I also became resentful because I realized that the clitoral information/definition was kept from me on purpose. This is knowledge that everyone knows, but no one discusses—that frustrates me" (Jennifer, age twenty).

These accounts show that the body has ways of knowing that transcend the general ways of knowing of the "mind" (Crossley 2006). Bodily ways of knowing unfold without the use of symbols like language and discursive information, or at least they can unfold even when such cognitive subject matter is only partially applicable and peripheral. The existence of silences and omissions—or of the general area "down there"—is evidence of the colonizing operation of repressive sexual discourses. This teaches us important lessons not only about perception, but also about sexual and gender politics. Indeed, the perception of iconic qualities—even when discourses inform it in subtle or tangential ways—is never context free and a-cultural. This is a remarkable realization. If sensations are never tabula rasa—that is, if sensations are never neutral recordings of stimuli awaiting definition—then a sociology and anthropology of the senses truly does offer an understanding of the world that is different from physiological and neuro-biological approaches to perception.

3

SENSUAL RITUAL AND PERFORMANCE

"Shit, where the hell is this place?"

"Hey, right there! Merridale Cidery, look, to your right," April—my co-pilot and wife—exclaims, just as I (Phillip) am about to lose my patience, long after losing my sense of direction. I quickly glance in the rear-view mirror; with no one in sight, I hit the brakes, abruptly shift down to second gear, and make a sharp right turn. Sharp enough for the road map, the wine festival tour map, the brochures we have been collecting, and my field journal to fall from my knees and scatter all over the floor.

"It's amazing how we drive the highway on the other side of this hill once or twice a week and it still took us for ever to find this place, eh?" I mumble to April as the tires begin to crackle and swish on the unpaved country road.

We are not the only ones exploring the back roads this weekend. The Cowichan Valley Culinary and Wine Festival seems to have brought a good two or three thousand people out of their homes—many of whom, directionless like us, seem constantly parked on roadsides hunting down locals for their knowledge of the area. License plates tell the story of a hedonistic pilgrimage that has appealed to the salivating palates of drivers from Victoria, central and northern Vancouver Island, the greater Vancouver metropolitan area, the rest of British Columbia, Alberta, and even Washington State. The Merridale Cidery is among the most crowded on this warm, early autumn afternoon.

"Oh, there's a spot right there," April alerts me.

Good eye. I park our Hyundai at the far end of a muddy makeshift parking lot carved out of wild blackberry bushes and shaded by young firs. With our hearts thumping in anticipation, we help each other collect the scattered papers and then head on the cobblestone path toward the main entrance through the dark red wooden building.

"Where do we . . . Oh, right there, look, there's a sign that says 'Tastings,'" I observe as I grab April by the shoulder. The place looks even more crowded than the parking lot led me to think. Yet the crowd doesn't seem to bother either April or this irremediably agoraphobic islander. We're far more preoccupied with trying to comprehend the norms of this wine-drenched social drama and our roles in it.

"Hi folks, come on this way, we'll finish this round of tastings in a couple of minutes and get another one started right away," hollers the server at us and another couple of wayward tasters.

It's a good opportunity to hang back and begin scribbling a few quick notes in my field journal. About twelve people stand around the counter in front of me. Behind the counter are two young women: one serving and introducing the ciders, and the other working the cash register. To my right is a larger retail room. To my left is a restaurant area, crowded with about forty patrons. Windows open the building out in every direction, allowing views of the farm, part of the orchard, and the steep, dark forested hill farther afield.

"All right folks!" A loud female voice interrupts my writing. "That was our last tasting for this round. All of the products you tasted are available for sale in the retail room to your right, and you can pay for whatever you buy right here with Cindy. I hope you enjoyed our ciders. Come on up to the counter, you guys in the back, and we can start another round right away."

Here we go, it's our turn. And it sounds like these are free tastes. Good for the research grant budget.

"Welcome to the Merridale Cidery, everyone, my name is Debbie and I'm going to be your host," Debbie exclaims, speaking a mile a minute while dishing out shooter-sized glasses to the fifteen or so eager men and women standing around us. "We're going to try eight different ciders today that are all made right here at Merridale and I'm going to be introducing all of them and answering your questions. Here at Merridale we work as a team to produce all of our products and we all play a part in every bottle. We love what we do and we love our cider just as much. Now, to some people, ciders taste very much like wine and even better than most wines, but some may find the fruity taste not to their liking. If you really can't stomach something, feel free to empty the rest of your taste glass right here in this cup, but still hang on to your cups because we've got more coming."

Debbie's script—conveniently "transcribed," as it were, almost word for word in the leaflet I picked from a table in the doorway—is as well rehearsed as that of a consummate actress, and our role and script are clearly those of a captive audience. Murmurs at the right end of the counter suddenly dissipate as she uncorks the first bottle.

"We're going to begin with our Traditional Cider. This is a medium-bodied, dry and effervescent cider that has been called the best English-style cider in Canada by Jurgen Gothe. It's the winner of the Northwest cider competition and winner of two bronze medals in England."

And with that, the curtains are officially wide open. Cider after cider, Debbie's frenetic act occasionally instructs us to "chew the cider," "hold it in your mouth for just long enough, but not too long," and "breathe it with your nose, but exhale before sipping," to detect the "woodsy," "floral," flavors. She also periodically introduces us to each of her co-stars: the "lighter, sweeter, but still very dry" pub-style House Cider; the "strong, sharp, rich in the flavor of full-bodied apples fermented to dry" Scrumpy Cider; the "sweet and rich Cyser: a blend of pure vintage cider apples and unfermented wildflower honey"; the "aged, dry and sparkling Somerset Cider with its balanced acids"; the "full-bodied still Cidre Normandie, fermented to dry, then aged in French Oak to soften the finish"; and finally my favorite, the Winter Apple—"fresh and velvety, with an aroma of baked apples and buttery brown sugar."

***

Wine festivals provide an interesting case study of the socio-cultural aspects of the senses and sensations. To taste wine would seem to be a very private affair, given how taste requires immediate individual contact between a taster and the tasted object. Indeed, that immediate contact—at least in the case of eating and drinking—depends not only on extreme proximity (whereas, for instance, sight and hearing can be experienced at a distance) but even on the physical destruction and bodily assimilation—through eating or drinking—of the object of taste. Yet tasting is hardly an asocial experience. From the social regulation of food safety (and consequently food flavor) to the sensuous components of feasting and fasting rituals, and from the association of local food flavor with regional and national cultures to the rapport between gustatory preferences and identity, taste has undeniable social dimensions. Wine festivals not only constitute an especially good example of this kind of sociality of sensation—epitomized by the commensality of drinking—but neatly illustrate the ceremonial aspects of sensation and thus the ritual and performative characteristics of the senses. As the ethnographic fragment opening this chapter implies, the senses are the objects and subjects of the *sensual performance of everyday life*, whereby "performance" denotes conduct, public behavior, and the carrying out of skilled, bodily action.

The study of performance is a highly diverse interdisciplinary field (see Bial 2004; Schechner 2002). For example, scholars interested in performance may focus on practices generally associated with typical cultural performances, such as theater, unscripted performing arts, acting, storytelling, film, drama, music, and so forth. Others may also study social performances, such as rituals and rites of passage, play, ceremonies, myths, as well as the performative aspects of mundane "social dramas" (Turner and Schechner 1988) and language and speech. This list is not, of course, exhaustive.

In this chapter we reflect on the senses and sensations as performance, and focus on how people sense in a performative manner, and on the roles that their sensations play in cultural and social performances. We begin here with a very brief explanation of why we treat the senses and performance together. Subsequently, we reflect in more depth on the sensual components of such performances as rituals, drama, ceremonies, myths, arts, and magic. Finally, we return to the wine festival in order to bring all of our key concepts and some of the relevant literature to bear on this case study.

First, it is wise to think of the ways in which people perform somatic work in the broadest possible terms. In common parlance, performance is associated with artistic expression, but we should not forget that performances occur in other contexts as well. Cars, for example, are said to perform well under certain circumstances and less well under others. Chemical particles perform in both predictable and unpredictable ways under experimental conditions. Sports teams perform well when they win; though they may perform well and still lose. Lovers perform well when they please their partners, and perform poorly when they do not. Stocks perform as well, as do workers who are called upon to perform a job, or students in an exam. By suggesting that people and material objects in these contexts "perform," we are essentially suggesting that they are trying to get a job done and that their success is measurable by whether they meet an audience's expectations. A singer who performs the national anthem before a football game is therefore not that much different from the team that performs plays during the game itself. Both the singer and the team are engaged in a type of action that is subject to scripts, rules, definition of roles, the execution of certain techniques for getting the job done, and expectations that stipulate whether the job has been done. To sense is to perform because to make sense of something is an action that is subject to scripts, rules, role definitions, and expectations, just like many other activities. In short, somatic work is performance.

As discussed in Chapters 1 and 2, a socio-anthropological approach to the senses rejects a facile binary opposition between sensation (as raw bodily experience) and perception (as cognitive processing of the sensations). One key problem with such a dualist conceptualization is that it treats the mind as an intelligent agent and the body—defined pretty much as everything except the mind—as the passive spectator recording external stimuli. Most sociological and anthropological approaches to the senses posit instead a fusion between the mind and the body. Indeed, those very two categories cease to make sense as distinct actors, as the body is *in* and *of* the mind, and the mind is *in* and *of* the body. An embodied mind and a mindful body "dwell" (Ingold 2000) within a world to which they belong, a world of which they are a part, and a world in which they perform their daily somatic work. Rather than conduits of external stimuli, therefore, the senses are work tools and "skills" (Ingold 2000) that are necessary for carrying out life within a social and material world. Understanding bodily, sensual, and mindful conduct as skillful action means understanding sensation as performance. It also means treating the work of the senses as an active, social, and often public form of action and interaction.

RITUALS AND RITUALIZATION

Ritual is one of the most common manifestations of performance. There are many competing ways of defining ritual, but in general most scholars agree that a ritual is conduct that is enacted "not for the first time"; it "has been done and said before" (Schechner 2002:52). Rituals may vary from highly stylized performances that carefully follow a formal script, perhaps passed on from generation to generation, to rather improvised and unstructured behavior that is still subject to "ritualization" in spite of its infrequency and irregularity (Grimes 1995). Ritualization may indeed be more comprehensive and less exclusive than ritual, as it refers more broadly to "the process whereby ritual activity is exercised" (Grimes 1995:60). More precisely, the process of ritualizing an activity—that is, of actively re-performing it—"transpires as animated persons enact formative gestures in the face of receptivity during crucial times in founded places" (Grimes 1995:60). So, how do ritualization and sensation intersect?

At their most basic level, the meanings of sensations are the emergent outcomes of ritualized memories inscribed into recurrent action. Memories may be conscious or not, and individual or collective. For example, for Tim Edensor (2003), the accumulation of memories of commuting over the same stretch of road over time has resulted in the formation of a familiar sensescape. Driving the forty-five-mile stretch from his office in Stoke-on-Trent to his home in Manchester means a lot more than just getting from point A to point B for him. Edensor admits he enjoys journeying alone on the motorway—the practice that many scholars have earmarked as the epitome of urban and suburban alienation from a hyper-individualized world of rootless nomads constantly "on the go." But, to Edensor, commuting on the same road week after week means finding comfort in mundane details and daily refrains, in familiar sensations and landscapes, and thus in dwelling on the sensuality and sociality of routines otherwise lost to distracted unawareness. That familiar sensescape is not only the object of his sensations as he drives but the biographical and narrative context that informs the ways he makes sense of familiar sights and sounds along the way. He writes:

> The sensual modulations of the journey are many and varied. Cones channel cars into temporary narrow lanes, which require concentration to maneuver, but then swerve back into the mainstream simulating the frisson of a fairground ride. Sometimes, the car dips toward the hard shoulder, banking down toward the ridges, which rudely disturb any reverie with a rapid rhythmic rat-a-tat-tat. Gusts of crosswinds tem-

porarily disrupt composure, even more so when large trucks pass by with a jolt instigating a firmer grip on the wheel . . . Together with the affordances of circumstances, particular occasions emerge from road conditions. Wednesday evenings, football season: The road is crammed with agitated fans hoping for European success, tense in anticipation and often gripping the wheel anxiously as the moving throng slows down. How far will a parking spot be from the ground? Will there be a chance to savor the pre-match atmosphere, have a pint or a pie, recalibrate the nerves, and settle into your seat so the spell of the car can fade? Wet winter journey: A foamy film of 10-foot high mist. White light shimmering on the road in the wet. At night, the tail lights bleed into the wet tarmac, suggesting a tropical sunset or a luscious fruit punch. The swish of the cars through rain and muffled sounds ahead. Summer traffic jam: On a warm summer's day, drivers surrender to the inevitability of a long wait. Some, frustrated, sit inside, drumming wheels and dashboards; others open doors, chat, lounge at the roadside. A sudden burst of motion ahead causes people to scurry back into cars, wind windows up, and start ignitions. Late night journey: In the dark, the illuminated windows of the houses close to the road seem to promise unparalleled coziness and warmth, convivial gatherings of wine-warmed intimates sharing animated conversation. The car seems lonely, an impersonal space bereft of comfort.

(Edensor 2003:160–161)

As this excerpt shows, ritualization is a skill and a tool that allows people to make something familiar, to deal with potentially difficult situations (such as foreign sensations), and with "ambivalent relationships, hierarchies, and desires that trouble, exceed, or violate the norms of daily life" (Schechner 2002:52). In the case of rites of passage, ritualization also helps in coping with difficult life transitions.

A great variety of rituals—of course, even those much more stylized and formal than commuting—are highly dependent on the activities of the senses and on the manipulation of sensations. For example, Howes (1987) describes rituals that emphasize the role of olfaction, and finds, in his review of cross-cultural studies, that people use manipulations of olfactory conditions to demarcate transitions symbolically from one status to another. The rituals he mentions range from odorizing by way of "smoking" a newborn child over the household fire for the first few weeks of his life, to the anointing of religious disciples with perfumes to express moral purity. According to Howes (1987), these rites of passage work at the logical, sociological, and psychological level to produce a feeling of liminality, a condition in which ritualization operates best (also see Turner and Schechner 1988). Manipulation of sound plays a very important role in ritualization, too. According to Jackson (1968), ritual sounds are of at least two varieties—human made and non-human made—and the two can be further subdivided in speech and musical sounds. All four types of sound resulting from this subdivision are used in rituals across cultures, by way of invocation, solicitation, or direct production. Certain rituals are also centered on the abolition of sounds, as in the case of many silence-based forms of meditation. In sum, the active enactment of sensory conditions is at the very core of ritualization. Ritualization, as Grimes (1995:965) writes, is "action thick with sensory meaning."

Ritualization serves to demarcate special transitions, but it also serves to give a sense of order to everyday life. Beside the example of commuting, one can think of the deodorizing rituals we use to cleanse matters perceived to be dirty or bad-smelling. In so doing, we assuage fears of contamination and reinforce existing ideals of cleanliness and moral virtue. In this context, Bichard, Hanson, and Greed (2008) have examined the rituals of public washroom users, and Dennis and Phillip (Waskul and Vannini 2008) have examined the everyday rituals of deodorization and perfuming typical of men and women in Western societies. Taste is similarly implicated in these order-reinforcing rituals. For example, Stoller (1989) documents that the Songhay people use the ritual of preparing a sauce so that it is thick rather than thin and watery to cement bonds among community members and between hosts and guests. The ritualization of sensation also works to outline life cycles (Almagor 1987), to express gender ideologies (Classen 1997), to create a sense of place (Imai 2008), to transform realities in magic-like ways (Gell 2006), and much more.

We will soon examine how the performance of somatic work functions in the context of specific types of ritualization, and highlight in particular the concepts of sensory socialization and somatic transformation. But before we do so, let us focus on the performative and dramatic nature of somatic work.

PERFORMATIVITY AND DRAMA

The concept of performativity has two primary denotations. The first has to do with the potential of language and paralanguage—and thus communication in general—to act and evoke action. Performance theorists in particular point to Austin's idea of speech acts (1962) and to its later elaboration by Searle (1968). For Austin and Searle, all language works not only in a referential fashion but also in a performative fashion, as people use it in concrete circumstances not only to refer to ideas, objects, and so forth, but also to accomplish social ends. As Austin writes, "to say something is to do something" (1962:177)—as is exemplified by the expressions we pronounce to marry someone, name a ship, halt someone, make a promise, and many more. While Austin and Searle dedicated their attention primarily to language and speech, others have applied their ideas to the study of paralanguages, such as iconic sound (Nuckolls 1999; Sullivan 1986; Van Leeuwen 1999) and the paralanguage of images (e.g. Kress and Van Leeuwen 1996). Their studies suggest that people use semiotic resources to achieve their communicative ends, regardless of whether they use abstract symbols, such as words.

For example, across many societies, the visual *icon* of a man exiting through a door is used to indicate a standard or emergency exit, and its display without the use of language directs people to move about a building. As an example of the communicative properties of non-linguistic sound, recall how competing runners immediately react to a loud bang at the beginning of a race. Or think of how we associate the smell of smoke—a sign called an *index*—with the presence of a fire. These examples show how semiotic resources other than symbols play key roles in social interaction, and how we direct our interpretive, somatic work at negotiating the meanings of these signs and acting upon them. According to Finnegan (2002), without these multiple sensory modes of interaction, we would not be able to communicate with one another and establish selves, cultures, and communities.

The second denotation of performativity pertains to the theatricality of human interaction. As Bial (2004:175) succinctly puts it: "something which is 'performative' is similar—in form, in intent, in effect—to a theatrical performance." Yet the term "performative" is preferred to the term "theatrical" as it lacks the histrionic character of artificiality and superficiality connoted by the latter, and therefore enjoys wider applicability. This second denotation of performativity is related to dramaturgy: the sociological theory of Erving Goffman and its followers. While Goffman never explicitly focused on the role of the senses in human interaction, his observations point to a social order punctuated by important sensations and non-linguistic cues. In particular, his remarks on the visual components of gender performance and identity (1979) and on the nonverbal dynamics of facework (see 1959, 1967), make Goffman's entire oeuvre a treasure chest of insights for sociologists and anthropologists of the senses.

The second definition of performativity reported above is also closely related to the manifestation of performance known as drama. According to Schechner (2002:110), drama is the domain of performance dependent on "carefully scripted actions." There are at least two main types of drama: aesthetic dramas and social dramas. Aesthetic dramas are generally prearranged, "less instrumental and more ornamental than social drama" (2002: 125). A play performed at a theater, for example, is an aesthetic drama. Social drama, on the other hand, is unstructured, its outcomes are less predictable, and its unfolding is more open to doubt, chance, and improvisation (2002: 125). So, whereas aesthetic dramas tend to be typical of the domain of artistic performance and highly stylized ritual, social dramas tend to be more encompassing of the domain of interaction in general.

Victor Turner offers a particularly useful conceptualization of social dramas (Turner and Schechner 1988). Finding that they are universal patterns of interaction, he concludes that they are set sequences of moves that people use to handle conflict. A social drama begins with a breach in the normal order of affairs. This breach is followed by a crisis, which prompts people to redress the situation at hand. In the end the crisis is either resolved or not. When it is resolved, the social drama ends in reintegration. When it is not, the social drama may either end in a definitive disintegration (such as a divorce) or give way to more redressing attempts. The senses and sensations play multiple roles in social dramas. As we will see in Chapter 6, somatic work often unfolds in concrete social situations as a form of social drama, beginning with a breach of sensory harmony (for example, as we hear an annoying noise, or as we detect a strange smell), an ensuing crisis, and a redressing action aimed at reintegration (directed at re-establishing silence, or locating the source of the strange odor, for example).

Now that we have explained the basic concepts and characteristics of performance in relation to the senses, let us take a look at some examples of performance.

MYTHS, CEREMONIES, AND SENSORY SOCIALIZATION

Myths and ceremonies are performative manifestations of the process of ritualization; in light of this, despite their obvious conceptual differences, the two can be treated together. A myth is a factual narrative that is often performed to recall together and share with members (or non-members) of a group how a particular society, certain deities, important persons, or the world itself came to be. A ceremony is a gathering—sacred or profane, special or mundane—of people that takes place in order to celebrate, commemorate, evoke, or otherwise perform rituals, play, and myths. The performance of myth and ceremony has important socializing functions: through them members learn about the foundations of a community and culture, acquire group membership, reinforce group bonds, and come to appreciate what makes a community unique and distinct from others. The senses and sensations play a key role in myths and ceremonies, though their role has traditionally been perceived as secondary to that of cognitive and symbolic matter, such as beliefs, values, ideals, language, and argument. But recently, many sociologists and especially anthropologists interested in studying myths and ceremonies have increasingly paid attention to their sensual and non-symbolic components. Performative approaches in particular have underlined the active embodied participation of both participants and spectators in the process of ritualization, and reflected on how the success of a ceremony and the strengthening of myth depend on the sensual dimensions of both individual and collective performance. Such active embodied participation can be understood as a form of somatic work; and the most obvious form of somatic work at play in these settings is what we might call *sensory socialization*. Let us consider some examples, beginning with the work of Paul Stoller.

Stoller's (1984) fieldwork among the Songhay of Niger shows that ceremonial sound has a unique force that penetrates bodies in deeply meaningful ways once one is willing and able to partake in that penetration. But neither willingness nor ability comes easy. During his fieldwork, Stoller himself was once reprimanded by an informant, Sorko Seyni, for being unable to feel the power of sound. At the end of a healing performance, disappointed with Stoller's insensitivity, Sorko Seyni sternly admonished Stoller: "learn how to hear, or you will learn little about our ways" (1984:560). To perceive the sensual dimensions of ceremony requires surrendering one's body to the potential of the senses, and often for Westerners this means acknowledging the blinding predominance that sight has assumed in our daily conduct and sensory order (Classen 1997). "The gaze of Western thought," writes Stoller (1984:560), "has seemingly ignored the dimensions of sound." For the Songhay, sound is the very foundation of experience, and Songhay ceremonies and myths unmistakably revolve around the expression of sound and the perception of its transformative potential. In order to feel the power of sound, Stoller had to endure a long and difficult apprenticeship, through which he became socialized to appreciate forceful sonic expressions, such as the sound of the musical instrument known as the *godji*.

Beside the Songhay, innumerable other cultures perform sound in ceremonies in ways that require a particular heightened sensibility—the outcome of sensory socialization—for its operation. In many settings it is often iconic, non-symbolic sound, that matters more than symbolic sound. For example, Ellen Basso (1981), studying the Kalapalo of Brazil, finds that ceremonial song texts are comprised of seemingly nonsensical descriptions of mythical characters. To understand a song ritual, participants would have to be aware of the stories behind the songs, such as the circumstances in which the songs were created. But because most participants are unaware of these stories, in spite of being able to recite the "lyrics," at a symbolic level, songs remain meaningless to them. Yet song performance within ceremony feels profoundly meaningful at an iconic level because it is the "specifically musical nature of the performance," the "pure singing," that brings together performers in the shared "experience of musicality," thus affording the performers "a privileged relationship with the special temporal–spatial frame of myth" (Basso 1981:288).

A sensory socialization is no different in principle than any other form of socialization, such as a moral socialization, a technical one, an emotional one, and others. But whereas socialization generally refers to a process of sharing values, beliefs, ideals, rules, facts, and emotional norms, the concept of sensory socialization emphasizes the importance of the somatic dimensions of adjusted membership within a society and culture. For instance, most of us are taught to appreciate certain tastes and abhor others. One of the foods that almost all white Westerners abhor is *T'lina*: an oily substance used as a condiment for salmon that is extracted from rotting eulachon fish. Learning to appreciate the pungency of *T'lina* may not come easy for most, but among the Kwakwaka'wakw of northwestern British Columbia it is not only a commonly enjoyed flavor but a substance that is appreciated as a symbolic mark of distinction because most white colonizers have historically detested (and continue to be repelled by) the grease (Jonaitis 2006). *T'lina* is traditionally enjoyed as part of the culinary feasts that mark potlatch ceremonies, which notoriously suffered throughout the twentieth century the repressive ban of ethically and aesthetically insensitive Canadian colonial authorities.

The manipulation of sensations is practiced in ceremony to express and achieve not only distance but proximity. Seeger (1979), for example, remarks that among the Suya of Brazil extremely loud, or otherwise low-register, songs that may last as long as fifteen hours are performed to solidify sibling relationships otherwise marked by a socialization that puts a premium on physical distance between brothers and sisters. While the fact that music is used to establish a feeling of community is arguably old news, the Suya are distinctive in that they achieve social distance and proximity by modulating the volume of their two types of ceremonial song—*akia* and *ngere*. *Ngere* is also the Suya word for ceremony, for song, and for music, as well as for the physical movement that accompanies musical performance. The Suya equate sensory socialization to musical/ceremonial sensibility with socialization to family and society writ large.

Seeger's (1979), Jonaitis's (2006), and Basso's (1981) studies of the sensual regimes of ceremonies are also important because they clearly demonstrate that the active participation of "audiences" in ritual celebration is crucial for the performance of the ritual process. Indeed, the word "audience"—which indicates a "listening" group—may be limited not only because it emphasizes hearing at the expense of other senses, but because it connotes separation from the performers. In his ethnographic study of the temple festivals of the Shaanbei region, Chau (2008) corrects this tendency and finds that people's active and embodied participation in ceremonies plays a key role in producing the sensory domain of performance and collectivity itself. By participating in a festival, people express the potential to contribute "to the production of the sensory event and the effect of the sensory event." Festival participants experience a "'sociothermic effect,' a diffuse psychosomatic sense of satisfaction and fulfillment resulting from having partaken in, in co-producing, red-hot sociality" (Chau 2008:488). Chau's formulation expresses quite clearly that ceremonies are not only occasions for the sharing of pre-existent sensory memories but also sites for the very production of collective sensibilities—a phenomenon that will become clear once we return to our study of wine festivals.

TRANSFORMATION IN ART AND MAGIC

Art is poiesis. The etymological root of the word "poetry" denotes this origin quite explicitly; but just like poetry, all forms of art depend on poiesis. Poiesis means to make, to bring forth, and, according to Heidegger (1993), to transform. Transformation may be "natural," as in the blooming of a blossom or the melting of snow into a waterfall; or it may be "technological," as in a tree becoming a wooden sculpture or making wine out of grapes. Along these lines, art, poiesis, technology, and transformation are closely related, even synonymous. Such a vision of art is obviously also encompassing of much ceremony in general. The complex singing techniques of the Suya, the powerful sound of the *godji*, and the other instances of ritualization and performance discussed above could very well all be conceptualized as forms of art, as much as of instances of technology. And a final analogy could be drawn with magic as well. When a piece of cloth stuffed into a magician's top-hat is transformed into a bunny, or when a wristwatch donated by an unwitting audience member at a prestidigitation show disappears into thin air, we certainly have magic, but also the application of certain techniques on the part of the magician, and the concretization of years of training and the manifestation of his or her artistic talent. In other words, all of these cases entail the making of something from something else: *transformation as poiesis*.

All of this matters because if rituals, ceremonies, myths, art, and magic did not *work*—that is, if they did not transform—they would be more or less useless. Or perhaps they might serve in communicating something to the social scientist, but they would lose the power of poiesis that makes them relevant to their participants. In the words of Schieffelin (1985:707), ritual "symbols are effective less because they communicate meaning (though this is also important) than because, through performance, meanings are formulated in a social rather than cognitive space, and the participants are engaged with the symbols in the interactional creation of a performance reality, rather than merely being informed by them as knowers." After all, think about this: are we interested in wine by virtue of the symbolic codes that inform its production and consumption and its positionality within a social structure and a cultural system? Or are we interested in wine because it tastes good and makes us feel different than we did before having a glass? To argue for the former is to argue for an overly cognitive and rational reality, as if individuals were treating their lives as a game of Monopoly played with rules drawn from social theory. To argue for the latter is a way of celebrating a sensual and embodied existence that is endowed with the power to experience (and enjoy) meaningfulness in its "qualitative immediacy" (Dewey 1934), and to make and remake these somatic transformations over time.

Art, poiesis, and transformation are at the very core of a performance-based approach to the sociology and anthropology of the senses. Take the sensing of flavor, for example. Rather than simply registering a stimulus, as Schechner (2006) writes, flavor is located within food and drink as much as it is located within the mouth and the context of consumption. Drawing from east Indian mythology and language, he refers to this phenomenon as *rasa*: "*Rasa* is flavor, taste, the sensation one gets when food is perceived, brought within reach, touched, taken into the mouth, chewed, mixed, savored, and swallowed . . . *Rasa* also means 'juice,' the stuff that conveys the flavor, the medium of tasting. The juices of eating originate both in the food and from the body" (Schechner 2006:12). In this sense, to drink a good drink, or to eat good food, is not an act of consumption that is separate from a practice of production. Rasaesthetics is a continuous performance, a process of poiesis that begins from, say, a grape springing forth to life and continues through various transformations until the wine is digested and transformed into fecal matter. And then something else grows out of that. This poietic, transformative process is punctuated at all stages by carnal, somatic, embodied experiences, and often experiences of *pleasure*. It is worth quoting Schechner (2006:10) again here, as the experience of pleasure is often forgotten by social scientists: "The snout-to-belly-to-bowel is the 'where' of mixing, intimacy, sharing of bodily substances, mixing the inside and the outside, emotional experiences, and gut feelings. A good meal with good company is a pleasure; so is foreplay and lovemaking; so is a good shit."

It is doubtful that we would continue to perform if we had no experience of pleasure. This is why the performance of somatic work is so often directed at the quest for pleasure. So, to be sure, to perform is to show, as ceremonies highlight. And to perform is to behave, as ritualization exemplifies. However, as Kirshenblatt-Gimblett (1999:2) writes, to perform is also "to do, to execute, to carry out to completion . . . It is about materials, tools, techniques, procedures, actions. It is about getting something done," and thus it is about taking delight and somatic pleasure in achieving one's purpose. In the case of food it is about making good food and making food taste good when one consumes it. In the case of art and technology in general it is about making something that is good, and achieving its poietic, transformative potential in the process of enjoying it, and in the process of getting the best out of it—irrespective of whether it is meant to entertain or to solve a practical, functional problem.

In sum, to analyze art (and technology) as metamorphic is to restitute magic and enchantment to it and to us (Gell 1998), to situate it within sensorial thresholds "where the corporeal meets the social, the somatic meets the historical, the cultural meets the biological, and the imagination meets the flesh" (Lepecki and Banes 2006:1). So whether it is the indexical power of the visual arts (Gell 1998), the sounds of the auditory arts in Africa (Peek 1994), the taste of drink at a wine festival (see the rest of this chapter), or that of food in the Indian tradition (Schechner 2006), performance is meaningful because it works (Schieffelin 1985).

PERFORMING TASTE AT WINE FESTIVALS

Wine festivals around the world offer the connoisseur and the occasional participant a rich combination of sensuous rituals, somatic experiences, and insights into the sensory orders that frame them. Not to mention many a good tipple. Determined to appreciate both the latter as well as dynamics central to the study of sensation, we decided to conduct participant observation during the wine festival season of 2008 in seven sites across western British Columbia and southern California. So, in order to revisit the concepts and ideas discussed in this chapter, let us now try to conceptualize the tasting of wine at wine festivals through a performance-based approach.

Wine festivals are *social dramas*, and all social dramas are *rituals*. In social dramas participants engage in a twofold process of action and expression (Schechner 2003; Turner 1974). In other words, they "not only do things, they *show themselves and others what they are doing or have done*; [their] actions take on a reflexive and performed-for-an-audience aspect" (Schechner 2003:186; emphasis in original). Social dramas, Schechner (2003:189–190) argues, have a generic performance structure comprising three phases: gathering, performing, and dispersing. To gather somewhere means to travel and then to assemble there. And, yet, getting there and entering the site is a *ceremony* leading us to acknowledge that the particular performance we are about to attend "takes place at special times in special places" and that surrounding the event are "special observances, practices, and rituals that lead into the performance and away from it" (Schechner 2003:189). In this way, the social drama of the wine festival is a ritual that also adheres to phases inherent in rites of passage (Turner 1969; van Gennep 1909): separation, margin (or liminality), and aggregation. Schechner's "gathering," in other words, is also the first phase of the ritual process—a separation that entails "the detachment of the individual or group either from an earlier fixed point in the social structure, from a set of cultural conditions (a 'state'), or from both" (Turner 1969:94).

Getting to a wine festival is therefore both a separation and a gathering that includes a somewhat exciting break in the daily routine of home or work. It involves making plans, reveling in the simple pleasure of a "Sunday drive," learning about a festival's organization, and a process of discovery (at least for those who attend a festival for the first time) of the location(s) of its site(s). Gathering—a process magnified in its dramatic scale by the itinerant structure of a multi-site festival—also assumes the quality of a pilgrimage of sorts. Surely it is a hedonistic and pagan-like pilgrimage built around a postmodern aesthetics of leisure rather than an ethics of duty. But it is nonetheless a liminoid phenomenon involving a break from sedentary daily life and a "rare bout of nomadism" marked by "preparations for departure," "collective experiences on the journey," and "arrival at the pilgrim center" (Turner 1974:167) where a voluntary communitas of taste is under formation.

Three sets of actors play decisive roles in the social drama of wine festivals: servers, tasters, and wines. Servers' scripts—like Debbie's—require them to welcome tasters onto the tasting stage (generally the area around a table or counter) and then to pour wines, thus introducing tasters to wines and to the basic rules of the performance. These simple rules are designed to "cast" (Weinstein and Deutschberger 1963) participants into their appropriate roles as tasters rather than mere drinkers. Indeed, the key function of these rules is to "defend the activity [of tasting] against encroachment" (Schechner 2003:12) from the habits structuring the practice of public drinking in everyday life. Mundane drinking in a pub, for example, imposes few or no limitations on the amount of alcohol one can ingest, the techniques one needs to follow for drinking, and the content and form of talk surrounding consumption. At wine festivals, on the other hand, by listing and evaluating the material qualities of wines and by outlining both the pouring procedure and the range of techniques available for wine appreciation, pourers set tasting apart from everyday drinking. In so doing, they allow a group of tasters-qua-spectators to become aware of the special quality of the performance writ large and the performance of the objects laying before them. As a result, tasters also become aware of their unique qualities as a group (cf. Schechner 2003:11–14). Certainly, while these ritual rules are organized around a pleasure principle, they are no less effective or forceful than rules laid out in more traditionally sacred rites.

One of the main manifestations of the forcefulness of these ritual rules lies in the expectation placed upon the taster to express an evaluative judgment of the qualities of the wines. After all, to drink quietly, failing to elaborate on one's sensations, and perhaps even to demand more booze, is typical of pub-like drinking situations where consumers use alcohol as a tool to combat sobriety rather than public tasting situations where wine's main function is to "objectify" (Miller 1987; Tilley 2006a) an art-patronage-like bond such as that between the pourer—often a member of the producing team—and the consumer. Thus, when servers introduce wines, they do not simply cast drinkers into tasters but also "frame" (Goffman 1974) what could otherwise be mere grog into an art object and therefore tasters into art patrons. Servers' power consists in "transforming raw experience into palatable forms" (Schechner 2003:30) through linguistic tools. Indeed, by introducing the wine, servers "actualize" (Schechner 2003) wines' artistic potential by making sense of consumers' otherwise fleeting, multiple, ephemeral, and possibly contradictory aesthetic sensations. Their "meaning in the making" (Dobres 2002)—their poiesis, as it were—is an artistic act as much as it is a technological act in that it "configures" or "scripts" drinkers and their practices by providing them with *taste vocabularies*: repertoires of linguistic sign-vehicles they can use to describe and evaluate taste sensations.

Performing Wine

"So, what do you think?" my pourer asks me (Phillip).

Here I go—I'm up. I am a bad wine taster. I can tell reds from whites. On a good day, I can find some reluctant certainty in the difference between sweet and dry. But that's as far as my skills can take me. This is not a problem on a normal day. I know what I like, and I drink it when I'm in the mood for it. However, a wine festival requires me to display a set of somatic skills by which the wine's own performance and the performative impression I make are measured. Now, to perform well does not just mean to learn to find and appreciate a material quality but also to become able to *make* a quality come to life through a lexicon of sensations and a script to be followed with care. With that vocabulary and script, I can speak with others in tongues. Without it, I can only try to listen to my own tongue. As an appallingly indiscriminate wine taster, I am painfully aware of these dramaturgic demands. As the pourer pours, I must listen. As the wine speaks, I must taste. As I taste, I must speak. As I speak, I must make sense. The sense-making of wine is far from being a private, Kantian affair moving from the tip of the tongue to the back of the throat. Rather, this joint somatic act begins at the very moment when a pourer and I enter each other's realm of awareness and ends after we have taken leave from each other.

"I like it," I answer after a pause. "It has a spark to it that reminds me of a white my grandpa's brother used to drink at the table."

"Finally, a Pinot that doesn't taste oaky," a tall, middle-aged woman standing next to me exclaims, overtaking the conversation. "I just had some Australian wines and they all tasted like oak. Let me try some more of your whites," she asks the wine pourer in front of us. He obliges. Gingerly pulling her wine glass back, she lurches her large, bumpy nose into the cup and whiffs at it. Then, lifting the glass with her right hand well above her shoulder, and gazing at the wine that is now dimly illuminated by the ceiling lights, she swishes it briskly before bringing it back to her mouth to sip. I hear a muffled swish coming from the inside of her mouth, followed by a complacent "mmh."

"No oak in that one, eh?" inquires the wine pourer.

"Not a hint," she consents, "and it's got enough legs to make me wanna chase after it all night long!"

Legs. I had to look that one up the first time I heard it. When a wine has legs a small film of liquid seems to hang on the vertical walls of the glass after swishing, then climbs down slowly to rejoin the rest of its body. Performing wine calls for expressions like this. Wines have legs, a body, a nose, and other human-like qualities that skilled anthropomorphizing tasters attribute to them. Other qualities include what Goffman (1967) would call face: wines may have no emotions, but their pourer's and maker's face is always reflected clearly through every looking-glass cup. Moreover, performing wine transforms the personal sensations of taste into communal qualities that may, then, be shared with others who possess the same sensual language, rituals, and discourses of shared meaning. This is significant. The other normative cultural constructs of the senses—smell, sight, hearing—have a patently communal quality; anyone close enough to smell, hear, or see can share individual and collective perceptual sensations. However, taste and touch are necessarily personal and "tend to divide one individual from another, for their enjoyment by one is either not shared with another, or is actually incompatible with such sharing" (Dewey 1967:222). Therefore, the dramaturgical ritual of performing wine provides a means for collective sense-making that allows people to enculturate material qualities ("legs," for example) as well as perceived qualities (i.e., a fruity or oak flavor) and combine them in ways that implicitly make the personal public (and vice versa).

***

Tasting is a "difficult art" (Peynaud 2005:72), but this is not merely because of the lack of correspondence between the paralanguage of sensations and the lexicon of symbols available to describe them, as Peynaud has remarked. The sense of taste is no neutral receptor of external physical stimuli and material objects. However, we sometimes forget that the technology of language does not have that quality either. The human senses are media "constructed out of the cross-communication of senses and things" (Serematakis 1994:7). So is language. And so is material culture. "Thus," writes Serematakis (1994:7), "material culture is neither stable nor fixed, but inherently transitive, demanding connection and completion by the perceiver." This aesthetic transaction is a performance, but not the automatic enactment of previous codes of high-brow or low-brow culture, or a devious process of impression-management for the sake of status-enhancement, or even a mere conspicuous display of social capital. Rather, this aesthetic transaction is the poiesis of an "amateur" (Hennion 2004, 2007). Talk about sensations is "poetry" (Fine 1995:245) and skillful transformation: "the making of something out of that which was previously experientially and culturally unmarked" and the simultaneous "involuntary implication" of the performing actor in a "sensory horizon" in which he becomes his own audience (Serematakis 1994:7). In other words, this aesthetic transaction is a creative "joint act" (Blumer 1969): an emergent, *joint somatic act* that bespeaks of the creative sensuous sociality of self and the transformative power of socio-somatic relations. Thinking of sensing as a joint somatic act, rather than thinking about atomistic sensations and individualized perceptions that record external matter and translate them into mental schemata and the register of language, allows us to understand the senses as conscious, reflexive skills we use as part of our dwelling-in-the-world-with-others (Ingold 2000).

In the context of a wine festival, a key component of our skillfulness is the performance of *somatic accounts*. These are creative acts: using germane taste vocabularies to pronounce our sensations, evaluations, perceptions, and aesthetic preferences. If we conceptualize a wine festival as a social drama comprising the phases of gathering, performing, and dispersing, then from the perspective of the festival participant the act of performing begins at the moment when our hand grasps a wine glass. While the nonverbal behaviors ensuing that act are important, the key component of our performance lies in the process of giving a somatic account. By giving somatic "accounts" we express aesthetic identities while "making sense" of the situation and the material objects at hand. When we give somatic accounts, we express the social, material, and corporeal character of somatic work. We accomplish this not by lies or poor judgments of our carnal experience, but by expressing the "sociality" (Mead 1934) of the embodied self and its sensations, and thus the senses' "capacity of being several things at once" (McCarthy 1984:108).

We give accounts by using expressions as simple as a "gustatory mmh" (Wiggins 2002) or by employing more elaborate vocabularies of taste. Accounts may be explicitly or implicitly solicited. They are explicitly solicited when others directly ask us to account for our sensations. A server who asks a patron "How do you like it?" is one example of that. On the other hand, accounts may be implicitly solicited when no evaluation is directly sought, but nonetheless an individual feels the expectation to express judgment to another. Wine festival participants are cognizant of the ritualistic rules that demand some level of spoken interaction among them. Thus, they engage in reflexive appreciation of the wine by talking with servers and other tasters, and provide somatic accounts even when no one asks them to. That they use the pourer's own taste vocabulary in their somatic accounts attests to the joint character of these acts. The word "spark" (which I used in the fragment above) had been used by the pourer himself in describing the wine to me. I did not parrot him by using it. He did not bias me by uttering it. Rather, by employing that word, we both focused our somatic attention (Csordas 1993) on a common quality of that wine, and through our common language our "aesthetic judgments" fulfilled their "potential for becoming consensual" (Fine 1995:258; also see Jackson 1983; O'Hanlon 1989:135). Thus, far from being a case of "monkey-see, monkey do," the novice's choice of relying on others' definitions of the taste situation "is a good way of anticipating one's own inclinations and of taking some guarantees, by partly dele-gating one's judgment to those who have other experience than oneself" (Hennion 2004:136)

To account linguistically for a sensation is not to disregard that particular sensation for the sake of saving others' face, or perhaps to relegate all somatic experiences to the realm of a handicapped crypto-language of the body. To account for a sensation within the broad domain of a culture's sensory order and within a particular ritualistic setting is to employ the senses skillfully as metamorphic skills. Understanding the senses as skills means thinking of them as "historically bound cultural agents, constantly being activated and repressed, reinvented and reproduced, rehearsed and improvised . . . in an intertwining process where the somatic, the physiological, and the neurological criss-cross the historical, the sociological, the political, and the imaginary" (Lepecki and Banes 2006:1).

***

"After the first sip, all wines kind of taste the same here. This place screws up your taste buds," a young woman tells me. A place like this—the Nanaimo Wine Festival tonight, but any other wine festival as well—*does* screw up your taste buds. Surely this is in part because of physiological processes taking place in one's palate. In fact, wine contest judges are well aware of this problem and have devised ways of minimizing its occurrence. But for a wine festival participant, the dramatic quality of an event like this also shapes how a wine tastes. It is the sensual hedonism that pervades this pagan ceremony: the multisensorial smorgasbord of a small ensemble playing jazz fusion far in the background, the aromas of oysters and candied salmon enveloped within the olfactory orgy of red, white, and blush wines. It is the haptic paradise of all-you-can-eat soft, creamy cheese bits endlessly leaping from trays to fingers to mouths, and it is the sight of continuous paths of experimentation and exploration that open at your feet as you determine whether you will cruise the tables sampling Rieslings and Gewürztraminers for the next hour, or stick to bold and dry varieties all night long. It is the harmonious struggle of habit and surprise, of the familiar and the exotic, of old and new calling forth performances of taste.

"A taste of our Pinot, madam?" I am suddenly snapped back to the here and now.

"Sure," she says, and her glass is soon wetted.

"This is a 2006," the pourer adds, "one of our finest years." The lady pounds the ounce of Chardonnay in one gulp and pulls off her brightest smile as a token of her appreciation.

"Thank you," she says. "I'm no wine connoisseur, but this is just delicious, the best one I've had all night. I would love to drink this outdoors, to have it with some fresh caught fish, maybe barbecued. It'd be perfect for a summer day like that, you know?"

That too—I write in my notes—would screw up your taste buds: a mild summer breeze at the end of the day spent by the ocean, perhaps lounging at a log cabin right on the water, titillated by a perfectly tamed barbecue flame. No, I am not romanticizing—I continue scribbling—I am just fantasizing about possible *pairings*; that's what wine-tasters do, after all.

There's a certain art to pairing. It is a seemingly esoteric skill: a dramatic act that masquerades as a mysterious elixir—the rather mundane practice of associating the sensuous qualities of an object with a precise context in which it is to be consumed. Just like an action movie is better when watched at a movie theater, or a symphony sounds better in a concert hall, a wine tastes different at a barbecue by the ocean, or maybe on a night out with friends, for a luxurious romantic dessert, or at a wine festival. Certainly, the contexts of consumption influence both how we make sense *and* how we perceive our senses. Nonetheless, pairing entails idiocultural knowledge that hinges on the perceived qualities of wine: the wine itself is like a genie waiting for someone to stroke the bottle. Pairing requires a willingness to believe in this magic trick, on the part of the human co-protagonists; to believe in the power of wine to transform and evoke multiple forms of sociality like a savory chameleon that changes the way it tastes. And yet, there is a dual process by which pairing is accomplished. It is not enough simply to believe in the savory powers of the wine; there must also be an equally important "willing suspension of disbelief" (Coleridge (1817), who also called this "poetic faith") which, as we have illustrated, not all wine tasters are able to accomplish. Coleridge noted that, in order to enjoy a play (formal drama), the audience temporarily has to suspend the knowledge that all is pretend—the obvious fact that the play on stage is not real life. Likewise, believing in the savory powers of wine is only one part of the art of pairing. The other part requires the suspension of doubt: believing that the wine has transformative savory qualities affords the thrill of discovery, sociality, and consumption. Willingly suspending doubt spares the pain of one's ignorance and personal taste preferences.

***

Wines and wine festival participants are linked in an ecological relation (Ingold 2000) and thus the sense of taste is based on co-dependence and co-construction. The flavor of wine is not determined solely by its physical properties, nor by the capricious judgment of each individual drinker. Rather, it is "produced" tentatively "during a "physical meeting" of the two, during a "get together" of wines and drinkers (Hennion 2004:140). It is within this context, within this commensality, that "we experience objects in relation to the community within which they have meaning" (Costall 1995:472). Taste therefore does not operate in a vacuum. In the context of wine festivals, wines are introduced to tasters within a structured setting that clearly influences the community of drinkers by way of conventions that shape somatic accounts, perceptual faculties, talk, drinking techniques, and sensual knowledge. The individual perceiver is not merely thrown into a world of unshaped sensations; rather, he/she "is introduced into this world by the people around it [the perceiver], and they guide it into this world" (Leont'ev 1981:135). The "activity of taste," in the words of Hennion (2004:136), "is accomplished through a collective which provides a frame, the relevance of the effort, and which guarantees results, accompanies, guides, [and] puts into words."

Taste as a co-production is inevitably "determined, trained, formed and deformed by its social environment" (Hennion 2004:138). The social drama of wine festivals is therefore a unique sensory order. A sensory order, or sensorium, is a society's embodied cultural model consisting of the "sensibilities that are exhibited by people who have grown up within that tradition" (Geurts 2002:5). Anthropologists of the senses (e.g. Classen 1993, 1998; Csordas 1993; Geurts 2002; Howes 2003) have shown how sensory orders as large in size as ethnic communities, nation-states, and even historical eras "educate attention" (cf. Gibson 1979) and thus shape the somatic awareness of one's world. But sensory orders that are as small in size as a wine festival can also work powerfully. At a wine festival, taste is circumscribed. Taste always "closely depends on its situations and material devices: time and space frame, tools, circumstances, rules, ways of doing things. It involves a meticulous temporal organization, collective arrangements, objects and instruments of all kinds, and a wide range of techniques to manage all that" (Hennion 2004:137). For instance, the expectation openly to express one's taste judgment typical of wine festivals consists of a "quotidian accounting of something routinely outside the quotidian itself" (Gallegos and McHoul 2006:177). Talking about our taste sensations is far from being a mere "nicety" or opportunity for "chit chat" (Gallegos and McHoul 2006:118). The nature of this simultaneously mundane and unusual performative act yields a uniquely acute sensual awareness. By virtue of this communicative expectation, wine festivals evidence the situatedness of interaction, of human bodies, of material objects, and of somatic and perceptual acts as social and reflexive processes. This reflexivity, this "pragmatics of taste," produces and magnifies "the performative nature of the activity of taste" (Hennion 2004:134). In the sensory order of wine festivals, therefore, announcing that we like a certain wine "is already a way of liking it more"; and by virtue of that, a certain wine "is perpetually transformed by any contact with its public . . . it is a performance: it acts, engages, transforms and is felt" (Hennion 2004:134).

The sensory order of a wine festival operates like other sensory orders working within different social contexts. As Fine (1995:246) argues, all "sensory judgments are grounded in social relationships, face-to-face negotiations, social structures, and organizations." Thus, to look at the sociality of wine festivals is also to look at the production of the materiality of wine, and in more general terms to "witness the production of the social" and the material (Law and Mol 1995:274). It is in this "relational materiality" (Law and Mol 1995:277) that taste as a social aesthetics resides. This aesthetic character of sociable interaction, notably recognized by Simmel (1997; also see De la Fuente 2007), organizes sensation and transforms the perceived object. The practice of pairing epitomizes this phenomenon. Pairing wines with foods and social occasions is more than a Martha Stewart-esque exercise in dinner etiquette. Rather, pairing produces different dramatic possibilities, which in turn differentially shape the ways both wines and drinkers taste. A particular pairing is but the performance of a unique sensory order. It is a performance that

> originates in impulses to make things happen and to entertain; to get results and to fool around; to collect meanings and to pass the time; to be transformed into another and to celebrate being oneself; to disappear and to show off; to bring into a special place a transcendent Other who exists then-and-now and later-and-now; to be in a trance and to be conscious.
> (Schechner 2002:156–157)

And, yes, ultimately it is a performance that screws up one's taste buds.

4
SENSUOUS SCHOLARSHIP

In 2008, my wife Michele and I (Dennis) conducted an ethnography on canoe travel in the Boundary Waters Canoe Area Wilderness (Waskul and Waskul 2009). At the conclusion of the trip we reflected on a number of things—not the least of which was confronting our own stench after paddling and portaging many miles on a hot summer day—as captured in the paragraphs below.

***

We lift the canoe on top of our Jeep, having paddled and portaged several miles this morning and well into the sweltering heat of a brilliantly bright summer afternoon. Water trickles off the canoe and down the Jeep, leaving tentacle lines in the dusty film that has accumulated on the automobile during the seven days it was parked in this dusty gravel lot. Opening the doors, releasing the scorching heat, I (Dennis) am struck by both the stale, hot aroma and oddly familiar smell of my vehicle's interior. Mostly, however, I am struck by my own odors.

In the open air you don't realize how bad you smell—something that is all too apparent when confined in our automobile on a hot summer afternoon where we are unwilling to open the windows and sacrifice precious air conditioning. I can smell our wet and soiled trekking gear in the back of our Jeep, but mostly I'm assaulted by the potency of my own bodily stench: a toxic stinking mix of sweat, sunscreen, bug spray, wet shoes, beef jerky breath, greasy hair, and three-day-worn clothing that still retains the smoky aroma of this morning's campfire. But an even deeper shock to the senses awaits me.

Driving down the road, I'm struck by the profound contrast in our modes of transportation. Twice Michele asks, "What are you thinking?", sensing that there is meaning to my pensive silence—something she would never have asked in the many silent moments of our canoe travel and intermittent portaging between one lake and the next. As usual, she is right. "I'm thinking about how fast we are moving," I answer. The narrow gravel and washboard-ridden road forces us to drive slowly. But still, forty miles per hour is infinitely faster than we have moved in a week, and the velocity is jarring. Our paddle and portage adventure of days now gone by was fashioned of slow-moving technologies and cumbersome bodily techniques that required conscientious physical effort and afforded plenty of time for sensitive observation. Not until this moment was I fully aware of how in tune I had become to the relatively slow and heavy pace of portage and paddle. But there is more.

"It's not only that we are moving fast. We are moving *too* fast," I say in response to Michele's second inquiry. I attempt to explain: "We are passing by everything too quickly to notice. You can't see the blueberries, the bugs, the birds, the flowers. It just feels strange to be driving through a forest and not able to really see it." Slow movement is idiographic and fast travel is nomothetic. Insulated by metal and glass, I am also realizing that "you can't smell the surrounding pine trees. You can't hear the birds, or the wind through the trees. All I can hear is the roar of my engine and tires on gravel." I slow down but it doesn't help. In contrast to our mode of transportation for the last week and the ways in which it structured my awareness, ways of seeing, ways of knowing, modes of understanding, and forms of being, I must now face the fact that we are *apart from*, and less *a part of*, the natural environment through which we travel. In a few miles, my awareness, ways of seeing, ways of knowing, modes of understanding, and forms of being will be entirely restructured.

***

Dennis's opening reflections exemplify the subject matter of this chapter, where we reflect on the sensuality of knowledge and examine the intersections between epistemology, methodology, and sensual scholarship. In the process of doing so we also offer further considerations on the concept that has guided us throughout this book: somatic work. In addition to being a useful analytical concept to understand the role the senses play in ordinary social interaction, somatic work is a valuable sensitizing concept for researchers interested in honing their *sensory intelligence*. In other words, we suggest that good sensuous scholarship is the outcome of somatic work, and that somatic work entails somatic intelligence.

But let us proceed slowly, and begin with historical context. Sensuous scholarship, it seems, is on the rise. Recent developments in and acceptance of performative, narrative, reflexive, impressionist, embodied, and descriptive qualitative research have paralleled an increasing interest in the methodological potential of "sensuous scholarship" across disciplines (e.g. Adams 2009; Bagley 2008; Crang 2003; de Garis 1999; Paterson 2009; Pink 2006; Sparkes 2009; Stoller 1984, 1989, 1997, 2004; Warren 2008). Sensuous scholarship has much in common with these research traditions and their call for an embodied scholarship, but it is also distinct from them. It generally refers to research, theory, and methodology that are *about the senses, through the senses, and for the senses.* Sensuous scholarship builds upon many of the themes and ideas discussed so far in this book. It pushes for the recognition of the meaningfulness of our somatic experience of the world, the performing of the skillful activities through which we actively make and remake the world through our senses, and the evocativeness of our strategies of representation. Let us start by briefly reviewing what sensuous scholarship is across a sample of social scientific fields and disciplines.

THE GROWING FIELD OF SENSUOUS SCHOLARSHIP

As an organized way of knowing and strategy of representation, sensuous scholarship is rooted in Stoller's seminal work on the Songhay of Niger and his subsequent reflections (1989, 1997). Disgusted, literally, by flavorless ethnographic writing as well as by his own initial inability—as a young ethnographer—to apprehend the sensuous dimension of the field, Stoller finds the need to write "ethnographies that combine the strengths of science with the rewards of the humanities" (1989:9). By advocating a focus on the sounds, smells, tastes, textures, and sights of ethnography, he argues for a radical empiricism that will "render our accounts of others more faithful to the realities of the field—accounts which will then be more, rather than less scientific" (1989:9). Taking his narrative lead from a serving of bad sauce, Stoller explains how the taste of bad sauce in a situation in which it was maliciously prepared, and later vomited by those to whom it was served, is not a mere colorful ethnographic curiosity. Important sensory events like that cannot be easily dismissed as meaningless incidents. Stoller finds that the fieldworker's traditional preoccupation with "big" and important topics and deep-seated truths causes him/her to miss those incidents—like the taste of bad sauce—that have great potential for shedding light on the somatic basis of culture.

Stoller's solution is to generate a new form of "impressionist and literary tale" (Van Maanen 1988): sensuous scholarship. This is tasteful fieldwork about, through, and for the human senses. It is fieldwork *about* the senses because it attempts to focus on a much neglected dimension of life: the realm of human sensations. Denouncing the power of sight as a dominating epistemology in the West, Stoller urges scholars to uncover the nuances of *all* our bodily sensations. It is fieldwork *through* the senses because it is the outcome of a reawakened and reflexive scholarly body: a body "stiffened from long sleep in the background of scholarly life" that now "yearns to exercise its muscles" and "aches to restore its sensibilities" (Stoller 1997:xi–xii). Finally, it is fieldwork *for* the senses: a kind of research that opposes the dullness of overly analytical, overly theoretical, overly formal, anonymous, and unimaginative scholarship. As he argues, sensuous scholarship offers a tasteful mediation of field experiences—through the written word or other modes—that occurs through mixing "an assortment of ingredients," such as "dialogue, description, metaphor, metonomy, synecdoche, irony" (1989:32) as well as sensations, the power of imagination and enchantment, self-reflection, doubt, and failures. Unlike bad sauce, Stoller hopes that this dish will truly appeal to readers' palates.

Since the publication of Stoller's original reflections, sensuous scholarship has grown considerably (for some methodological essays, see Adams 2009; Bagley 2008; Crang 2003; de Garis 1999; Paterson 2009; Pink 2006; Sparkes 2009; Stoller 2004; Warren 2008). Social anthropologist Sarah Pink (2006), for example, has situated the growth of *visual ethnography* in the burgeoning tradition of sensuous scholarship. As she argues, the contemporary attention to visual media of representation results from the new social scientific propensity to consider film and photography not as realist tools but, more modestly, as sensuous modes of representation alternative to writing, and not in any way inferior or superior to it. Pink's reflection over the potential of the visual to capture field sites, practices, and experiences is particularly illuminating because of her awareness that filmic and photographic mediations are but imaginative metaphors—not objective reproductions—for complex somatic realities that are virtually impossible to reproduce in their multiple nuances and modalities. Rather than viewing that as a limitation of the medium, Pink embraces the creative potential of visual methodologies for bringing to light sensations that are otherwise hard to evoke through other media.

The popularity of visual methods—driven in large part, arguably, by the growing availability of affordable and user-friendly technologies—has exploded as of late, but sight-centered approaches to research are not the only available ones. The growth of arts-based approaches to social research (e.g. see Knowles and Cole 2008) has meant that researchers interested in the sonic dimensions of everyday life can now tune in to a growing music-based (Bresler 2008) and radio- (McKenzie 2008) and audio-based documentary tradition (Makagon and Neumann 2009). Those keen on movement and balance can lean on the expanding influence of dance- and choreography-oriented strategies (Blumenfeld-Jones 2008). Those who grapple with three-dimensionality can shape their work through the lead of installation art (Cole and McIntyre 2008). And those who wish to combine tactility and visuality can weave new metaphors through such recently accepted research media as quilts (Ball 2008). Even food, at least within the arts and humanities, has been feasted upon as a medium for the performance of knowledge (Kirshenblatt-Gimblett 1999).

While visual ethnography and related visual methods, such as painting (Sullivan 2008), are among the most popular offspring of a sensuous turn to scholarship, other strategies have made great advances as well. In sports studies, for example, Sparkes (2009) has led a movement challenging the traditional disembodied approach to the sporting experience. Through *autoethnography* (for more on this, see Ellis 2004), reflexive ethnography, sensuous writing, and other modes of representation, Sparkes (2009:33) has pushed for greater recognition of the roles sensations play "as part of a vibrant and multi-sensorial ethnographic project." Among such other modes of representation are such practices as *soundwalking*, through which researchers tune their ears on the tonalities of the field and on the auditory aspects of interactions among social actors (e.g. Adams 2009; also see Hall, Lashua, and Coffey 2008). Walking as a strategy of "data collection" has also occasioned sensuous writing in the notable examples of Wylie's (2002, 2005) non-representational research on rural landscapes, and more generally it has facilitated the discovery of the sensual properties of kinesthesis (e.g. Edensor 2007; Ingold and Vergunst 2008).

Because sensuality is so much a part of the embodied and emotional experiences of place, it is no accident that sensual scholarship has found fertile terrain in human geography. Crang (2003), for example, has proposed that much potential remains for qualitative research in geography to be more "touchy feely" than it is, erroneously, believed to be. According to Crang, touching, and in general feeling, ought to yield work that is more deeply in tune with the material aspects of place. Following Crang's incitation, Paterson (2009:7) argues for the need to "find innovative ways to evoke or transcribe those underrepresented, unproblematized realms of everyday, embodied sensory experience." While these methods have not found a label as convenient as visual ethnography or autoethnography, we argue that they represent novel ways of engaging in *topographic and cartographic sensuous practices* and that they constitute good examples of the sensuous geography envisioned by Rodaway (1994). In sum, the growth of non-traditional scholarship across fields and disciplines has made it easier for sensuous scholarship to grow strong roots in an already fertile field. Academics and students who have traditionally been hesitant to write well and write sensuously—or use new media to do so—no longer have to worry about the acceptance of their work.

THE POLITICS AND AESTHETICS OF SENSORY INTELLIGENCE

Two additional aspects of the growing field of sensuous scholarship deserve our attention. The first concerns the power of sensuous scholarship to sensitize its readers, viewers, and listeners to the carnal aspects of social injustice. Writing about a brutal beating and its aftermath, Stoller (2004:820) observes that "a fully sensuous scholarship not only propels social scientists to reconsider the analysis of power-in-the-world but also compels them to rethink their scholarly-being-in-the-world." Integrating *social justice* as one of the main staples of sensuous scholarship is necessary not only because evocative and sensuous representations have the power to move audiences, but also because sensuous scholars are best equipped to analyze the sociologically significant ways in which dominant power orders regularly manipulate the "sensory regimes" (Stoller 2004:820) of their subjects' daily lives.

The second aspect concerns the appreciation of the unique sensuous power of *ethnopoetics* (Brady 2004), an aesthetic power that should be easily harnessed by humanist researchers interested in discovering the sensuality of the world. Poetry, argues Brady (2004:628), "opens up ethnographic inquiry to the whole realm of aesthetics." It does so through its playfulness, its self-consciousness, its counter-intuitiveness, its puzzling way of forcing the reader to question taken-for-granted realities, its conspicuous reflexivity, and its focus on signifiers at the expense of signifieds. Poetry's metaphorical potential is no mere substitute for the formal descriptive prose typical of dispassionate reports. It does not aim at reproducing and representing, but at creating self-consciously original impressions, at stimulating the recipient's senses to the reverberations of possibility, of magic, of emotionality, of storytelling. As a metaphor for sensual experience, poetry "finds the strange in the everyday, [and] takes us to another circumstance" that is unfamiliar to us: "Unafraid of its sensual immersions, its subjectivities, its mutual constructions of meaningful relationships, and deliberately fictionalized realities that 'ring true,' poetic rendering is more than another way of telling (writing or speaking). It is another way of interpreting and therefore of knowing" (Brady 2004:630).

Poetry is an enriching research technique—regardless of how "good" one may feel oneself to be at it—because it teaches us to be *sensitive*. And sensitivity is important not only because it allows our work to read, look, or sound better, but because it increases its pathos: its emotive potential to move and persuade. Poetry does this simply by forcing us, as writers and readers, to change pace. It follows a different rhythm from that of prose. Communicating in prose assumes a pace of routine, habit, and mindset—a pace that is sufficiently comfortable to allow (and even celebrate) speed-reading and to excuse distraction. By compelling us to slow down, poetry enables us to experience new sensations and rediscover familiar ones. For example, Dennis (Waskul and Van der Riet 2002) utilized ethnopoetics to evoke the dramatic pathos of chronically ill cancer patients—most were women, and most were confronting the later stages of the illness (of the eighteen participants in the study, all but four had died by the end of data collection). It is a gross understatement to call these circumstances dramatic, and precisely part of the reason Waskul and Van der Riet used poetry, rather than traditional data quotes, to convey what these cancer patients told them. By slowing down the reader's eye through poetry, Waskul and Van der Riet hoped to elicit a deeper experience of empathy and sensitivity. Take the passage below, for example:

> I think I am not so scared of the pain.
> I have access to palliative care.
> I am expecting there to be adequate palliative care.
> So, it's not the pain.

It's more the rotting.
It sounds revolting.
Rotting.
Ulceration.
Suppuration.
Being aware of your body
Failing in these ways.
Having an awareness
while I am dying
and dying in a state
where my body
is absolutely revolting.
I mean, *the ultimate bad death*.

(Waskul and Van der Riet 2002:498; emphasis in original)

Dennis does not claim to be a poet or a storyteller. Nor—as a healthy man—does he claim to be capable of "knowing" what it is like to undergo the experiences this female cancer patient is describing. But the point here is not to achieve certain objective or realist "standards" of empathy, but to seek ways to exercise greater if not deeper degrees of sensitivity. In a way, Dennis's poetry is to his prose what his canoeing is to driving his car: it is simply a tool and technique that he uses to slow down in order to become more sensitive and reflexive.

Much like we can speak of emotional intelligence, we can speak of *sensory intelligence*: a type of intelligence that involves all our senses and the reflexive cultivation of our sensations. Sensory intelligence is the ability to understand one's and others' sensations. It is the skilled use of sensibility to approach life situations. It is the ability to utilize one's senses as skills to manipulate and adapt to one's environment. It is the combined emotional, visceral, and cognitive ability to engage in somatic work. Without sensory intelligence, there can be no sensuous scholarship. Indeed, we will go further and suggest that all sensuous scholarship is a form of sensory intelligence. Insofar as that intelligence is the dynamic outcome of socialization, and of skillful performance, sensuous scholarship is indeed itself the outcome of somatic work. Thus, for example, a good ethnographer does not just automatically perceive the field as a set of external stimuli and then record it in their field notes. Really to experience the properties of a field is to make sense of it by mediating sensations through language. Sensations have a quality of firstness to them (Peirce 1931)—that is, an immediate, carnal significance—that is so inimitable by other sign vehicles, such as language, that to reflect on them always implies creativity, skillful mediation, and performative translation. In other words, the world as lived by and through our sensations is, in fact, inseparable from our creative interpretations and manipulations by which we render it.

This is hard work. Sensuous scholarship cannot easily tune in to the sensuality of everyday life. It cannot promise miracles or magic tricks. But through the work it asks of us, it can bring our experiences of the sensual world to life in their multiple shapes, colors, tonalities, textures, patterns, sonic reverberations and pulses, in their tastes and odors, movements and imbalances, fragrances and painful sensations. This is a project it shares with reflexive and performative writing (e.g. Conquergood 1991; Pelias 1999), which can poeticize life without pretending to duplicate it. It can give its readers, viewers, or listeners a way of feeling with us without necessarily being there. Sensuous scholarship can "celebrat[e] the multivocal, multilayered, and multivalent realities of everyday life" (Pelias 1999:x). It can build—rather than flatten—the elusive character of sensations, and it can allow for meaningful objects to participate in the world.

SENSUAL METHODS OF DATA COLLECTION

Now that we have hopefully clarified what sensuous scholarship is, and what its potential and challenges are, let us reflect on *how to do it* by examining in some detail how to design sensuous research. Given our limited space and narrow interest, we will not discuss here all the components of research design. After all, we believe we would not have much to add to existing knowledge on how to formulate research questions and how to select research sites, samples, or units of analysis. So, let us focus instead on the original approach sensuous scholarship has to offer.

The first dimension of this approach pertains to methods of data collection. Rather than suggesting that there are some qualitative methods that can capture everyday sensuality better than others, we want to convey the idea that *all* humanistic methods—from non-participant to participant observation; from more traditional to newer and experimental strategies; and from all forms of interviewing to autoethnographic introspection—can help us collect sensuous data. As a matter of fact, we find that the very expression "method of data collection" can confuse more than it can help. To think of sensuous "methods of data collection" is akin to expecting to look inside a box of magic tools and tricks. In actuality, collecting sensuous data is not an esoteric enterprise, and no method works like a powerful elixir. *Any* research activity has the potential to work insofar as we perform a bit of somatic work. So, it does not really matter *what* a researcher does; what is important is *how* he/she does it. For a handy example of what we mean, let us examine the practice of walking.

There are various types of walking: race-walking and marching, jogging and ambulating, constitutionals and saunters, parades and hikes. And there are various types of walker: one person sashays, another walks *lugulugu*, one tramps, another struts like a gangster. One is a pilgrim, another is a *flâneur*. The types of walking are legion. But let us not concern ourselves with these "whats" of walking, but rather with the "hows." As with all methods, it matters more how we conduct research than what type of research we conduct. As a straw man for our argument, let us take as the ideal type the habitual and mundane way you walk from your house to the bus stop or your workplace. This is the kind of walking that is easily done on automatic pilot, as it were. It is a mere way of getting from "point a" to "point b"; it is effortless, mindless, eventless. It is, in short, *insensitive*, or at least very low in sensory reflexivity. In contrast, take the experience of walking in an unfamiliar environment. Walking in a foreign place is a strange experience marked by contingency, uncertainty, and emergence. As opposed to habitual walking, it requires conscious effort and deeper focus. It requires us to be reflexive and sensitive. The same could be said of research methods in general. Un-reflexive and insensitive research—regardless of the methods one follows—differs from its reflexive and sensitive counterparts in the same way that habitual walking differs from reflexively conscious—or minded—walking.

The example of walking can teach us a lot because it is a form of *bodily* work. All sensuous data collection methods are bodily exercises in some way or another because they are dependent on sensory intelligence, which is a reflexive bodily activity. We do not mean to be exclusive; even those who are unable to walk can relate to the amount and type of energy that physical movement requires. All kinds of movement can work as exercises in observation, insofar as we abandon the automatic pilot mode. By positing the habitual as a problem—or by problematizing the habitual by adding measures of novelty, such as walking in non-urban environments (at least for city dwellers) or on unfamiliar streets—we are forced to reorient ourselves and seek a new balance. We are pushed to move ahead and take risks, to overcome discomfort and fatigue, and eventually to find our way back. Walking can also put us in touch with the materiality of our surroundings in its visual, olfactory, tactile, and sonic dimensions. By walking, we might even get hot, sweaty, hungry, or thirsty and get our sense of taste involved in the action. And perhaps by walking we will have a chance to meet and interact with our neighbors and make new friends.

Walking—in sum—constitutes a good example of the qualities typical of all sensuous methods of data collection because it is a *slow* form of bodily work. As Dennis's opening reflections showed, walking is not like driving. It is not like flying on the automatic pilot mode typical of behavior that is driven by habit. The slow pace of walking allows us to reflect and take notice of the unnoticed. Let us then take another look at what walking, or, to be more precise, portaging—as well as canoeing—did for Dennis. Later in the chapter we will examine in greater depth how he tried to represent his experience.

***

Travel in Minnesota's Boundary Waters Canoe Wilderness Area is much like the French voyageurs' journeys of two centuries ago: paddle a lake or river and portage to the next, camp the night, arise the next morning, break camp, do it again. Aside from travelers with trendy GPS navigation systems (rather disrespectful to the spirit of the voyageurs of old), travel largely demands reliable map and compass skills—the lakes, rivers, and portage trails are not marked; there are neither signs nor directions. The only signposts for a campsite are a primitive campfire grill (typically buried in rocks to provide shelter from the wind, making it even harder to spot) and an almost equally primitive hole in the ground that provides the most minimal luxury for fecal and urinary functions (assuming a tree or stoop will not suffice).

Along the more popular routes, campsites and portage trails are relatively easy to find because they are well trodden. In more remote areas, game trails are often indistinguishable from portage trails, while campsites blend seamlessly into the landscape and can be surprisingly difficult to find. The map will merely get you close, and the tell-tale signs of aluminum scrapings on rock will then be your best cues.

Paddling is relatively easy, if not leisurely, given reasonable wind and other good weather conditions. The canoe glides smoothly over the surface of the water with as little or as much effort as you wish. Michele and I use fifty-inch, bent-shaft canoe paddles that maximize the power and efficiency of our stroke. One hand grips the handle, the other chokes the neck: both arms extended, the paddle is thrust into the water and drawn toward the stern (rear of the canoe). As the blade plows through the water, one can hear a distinctive "schlooop" sound as a tiny whirlpool forms just off the edge of the paddle. Upon exit, you twist your wrists a half-turn toward the bow so that the paddle blade is horizontal to the water as you reach forward, make a half-twist of the wrist toward the stern, and plant another stroke. Immediately upon exit, you hear the dribbling of water off the paddle blade that, by the time you plant the next stroke, has dissipated into small drops. The routinized pattern is mesmerizing: twist, plant, draw, schloop, twist, dribble, dribble, drop, drop, drop; twist, plant, draw, schloop, twist, dribble, dribble, drop, drop, drop. In paddling, steady wins the race; just find a maintainable pace and rhythm—and an enjoyable one, at that. After all, this is *not* a race.

The paddler at the bow primarily provides momentum, while the paddler at the stern both contributes power and controls direction (mostly by the use of j-strokes and ruttering). One paddles on the opposite side from your partner, switching sides only to manage the light fatigue. Perhaps it is our many years of experience, but we find canoe travel refreshingly simple: we glide over the surface of the water with a casual feeling of flight. And thus was our canoe travel for seven days, across just less than fifty miles.

One of the most striking qualities of partnered canoe travel is how little we talk; and yet, simultaneously, communication is essential. In the canoe, Michele and I talk very little: a half-hour (or more) may pass without either of us uttering a single word. The silence is far from uncomfortable. It is, instead, quite tranquil. Besides, conversation in a canoe is not easy. Separated by twelve feet, and not facing each other, nearly every statement solicits the sometimes irritating but always predictable "Huh?", "What?", "Come again?", or any other of the common expressions for "I'm sorry, I didn't hear you. Will you repeat what you just said?" Long periods of silence prevail; you hear only the wind through the pines, the distinctive sounds of a paddle blade pushing water, drips of water as the blade glides over the surface, the haunting wail of loons, a rustle in the woods, an occasional screech of an eagle or hoot of an owl, and the more frequent buzz of maddening deerflies and mosquitoes swarming to suck your blood.

Yet, paradoxically, while talk is minimal, communication is heightened. While I'm controlling the boat from the stern, Michele must spot and make sure I'm aware of any submerged rocks, fallen branches, and trees—especially as I navigate the twisted bends of small creeks and rivers. I simply cannot see them, let alone avoid them, without her watchful eyes. But even in the calmest of waters, we share an ever-present harmony of communication—much of which owes to our many years of paddling together. Our strokes are synchronized; I can feel when she switches sides and I instinctively do the same. I know she's weaker on her right, where cancer so rudely claimed her breast and weakened her pectoral muscle, and I almost innately adjust the power of my stroke to compensate. I would struggle to navigate these waters with anyone else. Talk is only one form of communication, and the least significant for our canoe travels; a fact that might well be extended to many other dimensions of our twenty-one-year relationship. Regardless, the embodied and sensual experience of canoe travel is profoundly vestibular and kinesthetic. It has much to do with the senses of balance, equilibrium, and acceleration. Our many years of partnered paddling have culminated in embodied habits that assure our vestibular and kinesthetic senses are in balance—a balance that goes far beyond the mere physical feat of preventing the canoe from capsizing.

Portaging, however, is quite another story. You must portage to bypass dangerous rapids and impassable shallows, or to jump from one unconnected body of water to another. It is possible to plan a BWCA canoe trip without the burden of portaging, but you would miss all the true wonders of the wilderness. Many canoeists are desperate to avoid long and difficult portages, but Michele and I know that if we endure a couple of rough ones, we will reap the benefit of peaceful wilderness isolation. It is worth the effort.

Portages are measured in rods. One rod is 16.5 feet, so there are 320 rods in a mile. In our seven-day trip, we will portage a total of 1,176 rods—nearly 4 miles. But that is misleading in two ways. First, Michele and I "double-portage"—on each portage, we both carry a pack, then walk back so that I can portage the canoe while Michele carries the paddles, lifejackets, and other small items. So, in truth, we will actually portage 3,528 rods—over 11 miles. Second, the distance of the portage is only one measure of rigor, and not necessarily the most important. The terrain and elevation are what really matter. Rugged portages that involve dramatic changes in elevation simply hurt. The bulky packs carry the weight low on your back, and they are not easy to put on by yourself. Portaging packs is pure grunt work. The canoe is a more delicate, complicated task.

You portage the canoe on your shoulders, using a (hopefully) padded yoke. You grab the thwart and, in one smooth lifting and twisting motion, heave the canoe up and onto your shoulders. It is a rather tricky maneuver, and a pass/fail exam. But getting the canoe on your shoulders is just the beginning—next you face the step-by-step realities of carrying it. With the yoke resting on your neck, hold out your arms horizontally and grip the gunwale to keep the canoe balanced—a sometimes challenging feat when walking on zigzagging portage trails. Now walk a trail that often climbs up and down various rocky terrains. Over time, the balancing act fatigues your arms and shoulders and the yoke causes a slow, searing pain in your neck and upper shoulders (although, admittedly, once these muscles have been conditioned, it is hardly painful at all). Furthermore, with a 17.5-foot canoe on your head, you can see only about three paces ahead and nothing above three feet. You can tip the canoe back for a better view, but that is both awkward and more physically demanding, so you do it for only occasional peeks. It's hard to see obstacles, such as other people and partially fallen trees, so you are always at some risk of painfully bumping your canoe into them.

The portage trails can add to the pain. Close to the entry points, the trails are well trodden and relatively easy to negotiate. In the backcountry, however, they are wild and rugged. For much of our trip, the portage trails are no more than twelve to fourteen inches wide, extremely rocky, and littered with large, exposed tree roots. The paths zigzag sharply and are scattered with fallen trees or branches. The rocks are covered with slippery moss and lichens. Whether carrying a pack or the canoe, we must step with care. We size up each step and plant each foot with caution. Near the entry points, we can portage wearing our all-terrain water shoes, but in the backcountry we need the ankle support of hiking boots. Risk management is among our highest priorities.

***

Dennis's experience with portaging and canoeing is more than a mere chronicle of conscientious physical effort. By engaging in reflexive bodily action, Dennis realizes the resistance the world offers to his movements. His somatic mode of attention—to borrow from Csordas (1993)—reveals to him a world made by, and revealed through, his sensations. His tuning in to that world also shows him the necessity of performing his senses as skills with which he manipulates his environment, adapts to it, regulates his own action, and communicates with Michele. Walking epitomizes what is most interesting about sensuous methods of data collection: in spite of fancy technical terms, all forms of data collection—including walking—are but detailed, descriptive, reflexive ways of interacting with the world, as Dennis's notes detail. All sensual methods of data collection are reflexive techniques that grant us partial access to our own and other people's sensations. Whether we walk or talk, interview or take pictures, record sounds or administer research diaries and journals, all forms of sensual research are ultimately tools we use to elicit various modes of somatic attention. It follows that what is most important about sensuous methodology—or sensuous scholarship (Stoller 1997)—is the sensitivity and the reflexivity that these methods generate.

Every research project has different needs. For example, for our study on smell (Waskul and Vannini 2008; Waskul, Vannini, and Wilson 2009) and for part of our study on the sensorial appreciation of climate and weather (Vannini, Waskul, Gottschalk, and Ellis forthcoming), we found that writing encouraged some of our research participants to reflect in greater depth on their sensations. Thus, we provided them with research journals and asked them to record their sensations over time in written form. When compared with speaking, the process of writing tends to be slower and allows people to choose words that more faithfully express their sensations. Writing is also a creative exercise: it allows for aesthetically intelligent composition and more profound self-expression. Because of the greater anonymity it can provide, writing can also allow research participants to share experiences that would embarrass them in face-to-face interaction. At least, that was the case in our study on sexual touch (Waskul, Vannini, and Wiesen 2007). But writing has its limits, too. Not everyone is comfortable writing. And even if one is comfortable in principle with caressing a keyboard or grasping a pencil, writing can be time-consuming, and lack of time can make people lazy writers, or deter others from participating in a study.

Interviews are probably social scientists' favorite method of data collection. When open-ended, unstructured or at least semi-structured, interviews are a form of conversation. Because all of us more or less know how to engage others in conversation, interviews tend to work well in many contexts and for many purposes. For example, we have found interviews to be useful for our research on sensing the weather precisely because people regularly talk about the weather in everyday life. Interviews work well because bodily co-presence allows interviewees and interviewers to create a bond, to share common experiences, to reflect on differences, and to lean on the relational modes of dialogue typical of acquaintanceship and friendship (and bodily co-presence is not even needed—as the example of the interviews we conducted for our research on Second Life evidences). But, again, interviews about sensual topics can work only insofar as both interviewer and interviewee are ready to scrutinize their sensations. In discussing the weather with our informants, for example, we found that the lines of questioning that worked least well were those that informants found to be cliché-like and whose answers they took for granted. In other words, it was only when we asked "difficult" questions that forced them to describe familiar places and sensations, or prompted them to narrate, that both we and our informants learned about the quality of sensations. In short, it pays to make respondents abandon the automatic pilot mode.

Finally, we feel that participation and observation are the most difficult, but also the most rewarding, methods of sensuous data collection. As the well-known Confucian proverb suggests: "What I hear, I forget. What I see, I remember. What I do, I understand." By physically and sensuously taking direct part in a social activity—with various degrees of involvement—we learn from the inside, as it were. Our participation in Second Life, in the rituals of wine festivals, in the practice of portaging and canoeing, playing music for strangers, going to the movie theater, and walking around the neighborhood always felt like an enveloping experience: something of which we were truly part. There is much to be learned about the sensuous dimensions of participation and multi-sensory observation. There are qualities of sensual contagion that are remarkably transformative, and there are aspects of somatic interaction that can alert us to the limits of language and the immediacy of sensations. In addition, as recent research in social neuroscience suggests, learning by relying on all our senses will typically produce a more complex and multilayered understanding than relying solely on cognitive functions. When the entire body is involved, more brain structures are activated. But, of course, no act of observation or participation can work if we cannot communicate about it to ourselves and others. Rather than a mere neutral tool for reporting sensuous scholarship, communication (or representing through other media) is a quintessential component of research. Since we rely mainly on the written word to communicate our sensuous scholarship, we turn our attention to this medium in the next section.

WRITING SENSUOUSLY

A look at the value of sensuous scholarship is incomplete without discussing how we create our texts about it. Sensuous scholarship, we believe, emerges by combining the conventions of social scientific theorizing with those of the humanities. In simpler terms, we believe that sensuous scholarship is part showing and telling, part description and interpretation. In suggesting this, we do not mean to dismiss those writers, especially radical autoethnographers, who eschew explicit analysis entirely in favor of continuous storytelling. Rather, we are suggesting that sensuous scholarship runs the risk of missing the point without conceptual and analytical reflection. That proverbial point is about inviting our audiences to a double layer of reflection. The first layer is descriptive, not in order to claim that we are portraying reality objectively (writing cannot accomplish this), but in order to evoke and create in our audience sensations that evoke research settings, people, and the phenomena that interest us. The other layer links the ideographic with the nomothetic, private sensations with public discourses, somatic experience with sensory order, somatic careers with sensory histories, private recollections with collective memories.

In practice, description and analysis can clash at times, but along with Stoller (1997:xv; also see Brady 2004), we believe that "discussions of the sensuous body require sensuous scholarship in which writers tack between the analytical and the sensible, in which embodied form as well as disembodied logic constitute scholarly argument." Such dialectics, we hope, might temper the problems typical of performative writing identified by Pelias (1999:xiv): its tendencies to self-indulgence, and its theoretical and substantive irrelevance. Now, more than one reviewer of the papers we hesitantly submitted to journals over the years has lamented that oscillating between speaking through and for the senses, and speaking through and for the mind can cause pain to the reader. We admit our own struggles and want to share some of the lessons we have learned. These bits of advice may not work for everybody or for every project, but at the very least we trust they might help.

First, if we choose to write sensuously, we should consider abandoning the typical structure of journal articles, as the predictable sequence of introduction, literature review, method, data analysis, and conclusion restricts the potential of sensuous writing. Instead of beginning with an abstract point of view and a disembodied voice arguing for the usefulness of a research study, consider beginning with a descriptive scene that draws in the reader. We too are guilty of having begun papers with such exciting words as "In spite of the growing amount of research on . . ." Instead of such anaesthetic openings, consider flashbacks, flash-forwards, shockers, teasers, intimate stories and revelations, and a host of other narrative techniques that filmmakers, musicians, and writers generally adopt to entice an audience. At the risk of losing friends amid our colleagues, we find that film and other art forms have more to teach us than journal articles about capturing audiences' attention and stimulating their interest. And beside prefaces and introductions, we should also examine the potential of "messing" with any of the other typical components of research reports. For example, in contrast to the canon, avoid "giving away" the end in your introduction; place information about your research design and method at the very beginning (as part of your introduction), at the very end of a paper (as part of a "the making of . . ." type of note), or by weaving it throughout the text.

Next, we should blur as much as possible the artificial boundaries between the literature review and the analysis by blending those two together whenever possible. We should question the need to write conclusions that take the reader's attention too far away from the actual stories, sensations, and experiences we are trying to evoke. Moreover, we should integrate theoretical knowledge throughout the writing rather than devote a separate section to it—as if thinking was divorced from the senses and the physical body. Since, as social scientists, we typically experience the world (ourselves included) through sociological lenses, there is no reason to separate the two in our text. Also, we should try to adapt our methods to the field in which we are immersed, the topic we are studying, and the people with whom we are interacting, rather than to abstract and overly cognitive canons produced by somebody else, for other purposes, and in different locales. Rhetorically, we should attempt to communicate through a writing style that performs the principles of embodied representation and understanding (Ness 2004). Concretely, rather than using the declarative grammar typical of detached, universalist writing, we should use a subjunctive mode to capture the uncertainty, complexity, and plasticity of interaction, to convey how sensations and their expressions unfold and produce one another rather than pinpoint what causes them, to acknowledge the tentativeness, situatedness, and fallibility of fieldwork and somatic work, and to evoke a sense of emergence. We believe that these four strategies of sensuous writing (indeterminacy, performativity, contingency, and emergence) are key characteristics of all forms of embodied representation.

Take, for example, the writing of Heide Imai (2008), which clearly illustrates the four characteristics of sensuous writing we have identified. Her entire piece aims to reveal the interactions and sensibilities occasioned by walking in the streets of Kyoto, Japan:

> Crossing the main street, I follow the din: the periodic sound of the traffic signals, the siren of an ambulance, the deafening rhythm of music and loudspeaker advertisements reflected by metallic facades and plastic overhangs of modern, ferro-concrete buildings lined-up along the main street. Leaving the bustling atmosphere of Kawaramachi behind, I follow the silence and turn right into a narrow lane of the Pontocho district in which small restaurants and traditional ochayas (tea houses) are lined up. Walking further down the alley, I can see how a woman in front of me is watering the stone-paved space to cool down the air and to clean the place before new customers come. Captivated by her movements, I observe how the water is running down in rivulets, making a gurgling sound, before gathering in small puddles. After some minutes of being absorbed in the scene, I continue my walk following the sound of the lunch-break bell of a nearby school and the laughter of approaching people, echoing through this alley.
>
> One might think that the alleys of Pontocho are dominated by old, newly renovated wooden houses. Yet, most of the newer buildings are made up of fake, plastic facades, imitating materials used for the traditional facades of townhouses, such as wood and bamboo, thus producing a new and different sensorial atmosphere.
>
> Walking for some minutes further down, I encounter at the entrance of a small alley a street vendor offering drinks and food at his yatai or stall. Waiting to have a short talk with him, I decide to have his ramen noodles for lunch. It is noon, and the sun is burning, so why would you long for a hot, steaming soup? It might be another aspect of the Asian culture: even when sweating from the heat and humidity, you can still eat a hot, nutritious dish, provoking even more sweat before it cools down the body for a

moment. Trying this typical variant of yellow noodles, I realize it is not only hot but also spicy, watering my eyes and killing my sense of taste. (Imai 2008:334)

Imai attempts to paint a multi-sensory portrait of her experience by evoking sounds, sights, tastes, textures, and her feelings of heat and hunger. Even though we are privy only to her sensations, these are not merely ideographic. She links the flavor of warm soup to cultural taste dispositions, and critically scrutinizes the building facades in light of the socio-cultural dimensions of architecture. Moreover, Imai's writing is obviously reflexive: "I" is speaking, rather than the impersonal verb typical of positive science, or the royal "we" connoting an alleged commonality of experience.

Imai's writing is also uncertain and plastic. Notice how her walking trajectory is not set in advance; and we are merely walking alongside her, not knowing where to go next. She presents her own sensations to us in a non-representational way; notice how she weaves complex layers of the contradictory "stimuli" that comprise Pontocho. She does not present it as the epitome of anything (e.g. traditional Japan, modern Kyoto, etc.) but as a complex entity on its own. Imai's writing is also contingent and thus her experience unfolds as subject to natural change. After all, it is only because she is waiting to have a short talk with a street vendor that she decides on the spur of the moment to buy his noodles. Finally, her writing evokes a sense of process, evidenced by temporal markers ("it is noon") and by a trajectory through which she moves. Similar characteristics could be drawn out from Dennis's writing.

Also written in the first-person singular, Dennis chronicles his effort and describes movement not as an accomplished fact but as a struggle. In this way his writing is subjunctive and indeterminate. His experience opens the writing and the reading to his multiple kinesthetic sensations, and his own movement through place opens up the field to new experiences, such as smells, sights, and haptic domains. In this sense his writing is performative: it brings a reality to life rather than explaining it away as a by-product of causes determining his actions. Also, Dennis's writing and experiences are contingent. By admitting his fallibility in verbally communicating with Michele, Dennis demonstrates how everyday sensory worlds are ephemeral, fragile, tentative, unpredictable, and demanding. Finally, through the very feeling of moving through the time–space of the Boundary Waters Canoe Wilderness Area, Dennis evokes a sense of emergence. His story literally invites us aboard his canoe and guides us through the wilderness area as if we were there with him. Much too often traditional qualitative research claims to study emergence without also being emergent. Thus, instead of serving us "themes," "codes," and "categories," Dennis's story makes us move alongside him, and his use of the present tense enhances the quality of indeterminacy. We do not know what is going to happen next.

REFLEXIVITY AS SOMATIC WORK

Sensuous research produces embodied knowledge. So much has been written lately on the topic of bodily ways of knowing, embodied writing, embodied ethnography, and related themes that we will not attempt even a quick review. Here, we want to highlight how sensuous scholarship builds on the reflexive turn in the social sciences. Reflexivity, simply put, is the activity of turning back on oneself, or the action of taking the role of the other in examining oneself. To be reflexive is to put ourselves in somebody else's shoes and imagine how this other perceives us. In the context of qualitative research, reflexivity means examining our assumptions, rapport with informants, choice of topic, research questions, methods, paradigmatic choices, analytic strategies, and writing styles. It means coming to terms with how and why the research we do is . . . "so us!" It also means examining how our biography shapes what we know and want to know. For example, our gender, age, ethnicity, subcultural identity, class, and region of residence shape what we know, how we think and feel, and how we are embodied. Being reflexive also means being able to take into account the presence we establish in the field through our (always embodied) methods. In sum, reflexivity means seriously taking into consideration the researcher as a mindful body; a body that is obviously and inevitably present in the research process.

In the context of sensuous writing and embodied research, reflexivity means that we must write in the first-person singular. It is only by doing so that we can take responsibility for our own writing and analysis. This is why we have identified the authors of all the ethnographic excerpts we provide in this book—the products of three different bodies. But beside writing in the first-person singular, reflexivity also means reflecting on the relationship between singularity and plurality. As much as we are individuals with our own unique sensations, emotions, ways of thinking, values, and bodies, we are also people who share many cultural characteristics with one another. For example, we share a language, a continent, intellectual dispositions, and values. There are also key differences among us—for example, English is Dennis's native tongue but not Simon's or Phillip's. And despite residing on the same continent, we live in very different geographical, socio-political, and climatic milieus. Simon must adapt to the brutal Las Vegas desert heat, Dennis has to brave the cold climate of Minnesota every winter, whereas Phillip must adjust to the rain and cloudy skies of Canada's West Coast. These are not unimportant details of our lives that should best be relegated to footnotes. These—and many other characteristics of our individual lives—are the matter of our *habits*, our *ways of life*, our embodiment, consciousness, and *culture*. A sociological and anthropological study of the senses and sensation must necessarily take into account individual idiosyncrasies in the context of pluralities such as these.

To be reflexive about the senses and sensations means to oscillate between idiosyncratic bodily experiences and collective experiences that have cemented in trans-situational social norms, shared values, common practices, rituals, and ways of knowing. These collective experiences make up sensory orders, somatic rules, and other plural ways of making sense of the world that we—as researchers of the senses—must always take into account as we conceptualize and analyze our own and other people's experiences. Practically, it means oscillating between the situation at hand and the wider context in order to make sense of the present situation. But it also means leaping back and forth—in the exercise typical of hermeneutic analysis—between foreground and background, between the description of the here and now and its contextualization and interpretation, and therefore between our empirical material and our theoretical concepts. As we mentioned earlier, this oscillation can be problematic at times. Switching voices—from the poetic to the theoretical—can be awkward and disorienting. But if we understand that to reflect on ours or others' sensations is the key of any interpretive act, then we should feel a bit more confident in utilizing a theoretical voice that speaks not only through and to the mind, but also through and to the senses.

We conclude this chapter with an example taken from John Wylie's (2005) reflection on walking on a path on the southwest coast of England. His words are descriptive and interpretive in a seamless way. He does not need to switch off his descriptive voice and turn on his theoretical voice abruptly. The passage is smooth, continuous, and effortless because his thoughts arise from his embodied experiences, from his presence in the field, and from his sensations.

> The pressure of the Path forced me to my feet. About five minutes' walk south from Hartland Point, having meandered through a series of sleepy, hedged lanes, it curved left, and I found myself, in an instant as it seems in memory, standing before a resplendent landscape, the best for days: the view looking south into the Smoothlands valley and the coastline carried far beyond. The shelving promontory is marked on the maps as Damehole Point, the first of a series of headlands knifing out into the waves. And behind the apparently nameless, faceless cliff, gathering the sunlight and becoming the configuring centre of the landscape, there is the "strange, lonely, wild little valley" (Tarr 1996:106) of Smoothlands. Lofty scenes are commonly supposed to inspire lofty thoughts. This one seemed peculiarly affecting and archetypal. It looked somehow too good to be true, as if it had been digitally enhanced and cleaned. It was spectacular: I was all eyes. The quotidian rhythm of walking, connoting an understanding of landscape as a milieu of corporeal immersion, is counterposed by a visionary moment of drama and transfiguration. The ambit of landscape seems to range all the way from humdrum occupancy to sublime optics. But the latter register emerges from Western visual cultures extensively critiqued for their objectification of externality and centring of the gazing subject. Sublime experience is predicated upon an initial fracture that places observer and observed on either side of an abyss. And just as the sublime

> beholder dissolves in dreadful delight, so he or she simultaneously undergoes an energizing apotheosis: the event of vision begins and ends with a cleaving apart of subject and world. In this way the poetic apprehension of dramatic natural scenery clarifies within a spectatorial epistemology, one which positions landscape as a slice of external reality seen from the perspective of a detached subject, a subject whose gaze is variously invested with notions of control, separation, authority and voyeuristic judgement. If corporeal rhythms immerse, then visual events, however dramatic and unforeseen, distance.
>
> (Wylie 2005:242)

Wylie's sensuous writing works because his interpretation is neither overly cognitive nor implied. It neither hits you on the top of your head like a hammer—as if to say: "Now, here comes the theory"—nor forces you to guess what he is hiding. Wylie's writing works as a form of sensuous scholarship because, at least in our mind, it is a form of somatic work. Somatic work is not just an activity that "research subjects" do. It is not a process that simply describes how "people out there" make sense of their worlds in social and embodied ways. Somatic work is also an activity that we, as sensuous researchers, must perform. We accomplish it first by focusing on sensations—which are some of the most private and taken-for-granted experiential phenomena of individual and social life. We must hone our sensitivity, our ability to apprehend the sensuous properties of our data, much like we invite our informants to do when we ask them a question. Second, in evoking these lifeworlds of experience through words, images, or sounds, we must first "translate" the qualitative immediacy of sensations into metaphors. This is not an automatic task. It requires deploying representation technics and techniques; it demands skill, and constitutes a creative act, a form of poiesis. And third, in understanding sensory lifeworlds, we use abstract ideas and concepts much like our informants utilize somatic rules to make sense of their experiences, to oscillate between singularity and plurality. While these suggestions will not guarantee the success of sensuous scholarship as a post-traditional practice of representation, they will go a long way toward making our descriptive and interpretive work less anaesthetic.

Part II

Doing Sensory Research

5

THE SENSUOUS SELF AND IDENTITY

The sound of barking dogs follows me (Simon) like bad karma, and my reaction is often volatile. I am not sure why. It may have started when I was five or six years old. I would come home from school, open the heavy metal door to our apartment building, and inadvertently provoke the concierge's white French poodle to run out of her apartment and jump too close to my face, snapping and barking violently. It often took the concierge a long time finally to call her dog off. Ever since then, barking dogs have enraged me.

When we moved to our first house in Las Vegas, our neighbors' dogs—which were left outside in temperatures approaching 115 degrees Fahrenheit—would bark endlessly throughout the day and night. Unsurprisingly, these neighbors ignored my initial polite suggestions that they bring their dogs inside, then my subsequent frustrated requests that they do so, and finally my threats to call Animal Protection if they failed to comply. Once, storming angrily outside in the middle of the night, I slammed my front door so violently that its window smashed into a thousand pieces. The next year, we decided to move into a gated community whose regulations are comprehensive and unambiguous with regard to barking dogs. Unfortunately, my new neighbor did not seem to understand them, as he too had an enormous dog, which was left outside all day long in the hot Las Vegas sun and would bark aggressively whenever we would step on our back patio or let our cats—Minou and Fidel—out for a stroll around the neighborhood. As repeated verbal and written interventions on my part failed to obtain his compliance with the sonic order of our community, one day, unable to take it any more, I brought my electric guitar and amplifier out on the back patio, turned the amp's distortion knob to its maximum power, and unleashed a loud, screeching, and dissonant solo that must have forever changed his appreciation of the sonic terror I could unleash, literally, from my fingertips.

My sensuous identity is partly responsible for these visceral reactions to what I perceive as too loud a voice or a noise. For as long as I can remember, my parents frowned on both, but for different reasons. For my father, calm and even voices distinguished us (the well groomed) from them (the uncouth), the well educated from the uncultured. Years later, I still catch myself judging acquaintances' speech with that same and now unacceptable equation. But while such distinctions sound unmistakably classist, carelessness with voice and the sounds we produce is also frowned upon in the Buddhist and other traditions. Sound is sacred and significant. In the beginning was the Word and Om is the sound of the world. Loud noises and voices are often used as tools of warfare, intimidation, and torture—from the walls of Jericho to the cells of Guantanamo. My mother associates loud voices with violence and terror. As she often tells me, even after all these years, she can never forget listening, terrified, to Hitler's vociferous rants broadcast over the radio when she was young.

Her cousin, the soft-spoken and easygoing Erwin—an Auschwitz survivor—was surprisingly intolerant of loud voices. I will never forget the tourist boat ride around Manhattan I took with him the first time I came to America. Sitting on uncomfortable benches on the top deck, his explanations of the various landmarks suddenly stopped as his face became noticeably irritated and anxious. "Something wrong?" I asked him. He did not answer but stood up and strode with uncommon resolve toward a group of young German tourists speaking loudly as they were trying to make themselves heard over the roaring boat engine. I do not know what he told them, but they became immediately silent. "Those Germans," he said, sitting next to me again, "they always have to shout. Makes me sick." Years later, I found that we can indeed reduce the noxious effects of adrenalin triggered by loud noise by physically intervening at the source.

***

"[M]an (the worker)," Karl Marx (1967:292) famously wrote, "feels that he is acting freely only in his animal functions—eating, drinking, and procreating, or at most in his shelter and finery—while in his human functions he feels only like an animal. The animalistic becomes the human and the human the animalistic." Marx's point is understandable in the broader context of his conceptual argument and framework. Humans, however, are no ordinary animals. Our so-called "animal functions" are just as potentially creative, expressive, and reflexive as our "human functions." The human animal is just as capable of cultivating and enculturating the aesthetic and sensuous properties of speaking (as our opening example illustrates) but also eating, drinking, and procreating as we can in our language, labor, art, or any other uniquely human activity. That is why we may refine our tastes in fine cuisine (if not develop our culinary skills), acquire the aesthetics for fine wine, cultivate a sonic appreciation of silence, practice tantric sex, or merely invest in any of the plethora of choices we have in the burgeoning market of books, magazines, or DVDs that promise to make us better lovers. The human animal is both subject and object of sensual experience, partly because of the necessarily active and reflexive ways we make sense of the world and partly because sensual experience intersects with self and identity work.

An evening of candles, roses, champagne, satin sheets, delicate touches, soft music, and whispered sweet nothings does more than merely "set the mood." This kind of sensual orchestration may help stage, incite, or reinforce emotional states but also reflects and brings forth one's identity as a lover—one with intentions (and plans) to *be* a lover. The music we listen to not only reflects and shapes our mood and listening preferences (DeNora 2000) but is part-and-parcel of significant forms of identity work that, perhaps, are most salient among musical subcultures (Goths, punks, emos, Deadheads, etc.) but might be equally relevant for most of us in subtler ways. Notice how the sounds in our environment (as Simon so vividly narrated) or the smell of certain objects (as we will soon see) can bring forth identities—past and present—that not only remind us of times, people, and places but help narrate a self over time: fresh-baked cookies, Corona with a twist of lime, freshly brewed coffee, pumpkin pie, fire-roasted marshmallows on a stick, homemade bread—to name a few of the smells and tastes that are commonly associated with specific people and places that have shaped our selves and identities over time. Selfhood, subjectivity, personhood, and identity—all the key ways in which the human animal is both subject and object of reflexive sensual experience, and a very special kind of animal, are the subject of this chapter.

The embodied self is both the material basis and reflexive outcome of perceived sensations and sense-making practices. In this way, sensations and sense-making body forth a *sensuous self*: a performative, reflexive, perceptive, intentional, indeterminate, emergent, embodied being-in-the-world. Just as interactionists conceive of the self as an empirical and agentic product of reflexive action, experience, and performance, so too the sensuous self emerges in somatic experience, fashioned by the practices and rituals through which we gain a sense of ourselves and the sensory order in which we live. The practices and rituals of the sensuous self abound in everyday life. These performances are often unrehearsed and fully improvised, yet carefully scripted by the nature of habit, memory, and past sensations, both dreaded and preferred. As a whole, this personal heritage constitutes a *somatic career*: a sensuous personal and social identity by which we recognize ourselves across situations and by which others recognize us.

Our key concern in this chapter—as it will be in all the subsequent chapters—is to deepen our understanding of sensory dynamics by drawing from our own research in depth. For this chapter, we mostly draw from our studies on olfaction and nostalgia. The smell of certain odors has a remarkable power to remind us of specific times, people, and places that are significant sites for self and identity work. We begin by laying out the conceptual foundations of *sensuous subjectivity* and then move on to reflecting on people's sensory experiences in these domains.

THE SENSUOUS SELF

Researchers of the senses speak of selfhood in different ways. Rice (2003), for example, speaks of "soundselves" in regards to how patients in the Edinburgh Royal Infirmary relate to the soundscapes of the hospital. As Rice (2003:4) explains:

> The sounds of medical practices, equipment and technology punctuate and pervade hospital life, and have been endowed with particular significance by many of the patients . . . They express an understanding that the soundscape is produced through the enactment of a code of medical practice (which anthropologists know as biomedicine) which requires them to be the passive recipients of medical attention, the objects of medical techniques, and accepting of certain systems of control.

Whereas Rice invokes the notion of subjects and objects of institutional practice to discuss soundselves, we conceptualize selfhood by emphasizing creation and somatic accomplishment. For us, subjectivity is not merely a space where power inscribes itself, but rather the material basis as well as the reflexive and interactional outcome of perceived sensations and active sense-making practices. Conceptualizing the self as a sensuous process emphasizes the somatic dimensions of existence and the "fusion of the intelligible and the sensible" (Stoller 1997:xv).

Symbolic interactionists posit self as emergent in the dual processes of knower and known—what Mead (1934) identified as a form of minding, or internalized *conversation.* We do not disagree with this principle but merely suggest that, in addition, through our *somatic* perceptions of the world, we gather immediate awareness of its sensual qualities and potential for meaning (Dewey 1934). Thus, the self is not only a knowing subject and the object of symbolic (and largely linguistic) knowledge, but also and more precisely a feeling and sensing subject and the object of somatic experience. Perception *is* knowledge (Dewey 1934; Merleau-Ponty 1962), and reflexive sensations accumulated over time and place constitute a somatic history and a sense of emplacement (Rodaway 1994). Somatic self-awareness, this cache of sensuous experience, generates the sensuous self. The sensuous self is thus sensing and sensed: at once emergent and conventional, subject and object, individual and social, body-within-mind, and mind-within-flesh. Thus, the lens of somatic work allows us to conceptualize selfhood as sensing and sensed—both by self and by others; a sensuous self that is a reflexive object of one's own somatic action. Somatic work is to the sensuous self what minding and internal conversation are to traditional Meadian (1934) conceptions of self-as-linguistic-product.

Owing to our pragmatist roots, we conceive self not as a metaphysical essence, but as a grounded empirical concept—an agentic product of action, experience, and performance. Likewise, the sensuous self is emergent from somatic experience. More specifically, we fashion sensuous selves in rituals through which we gain a sense of ourselves and the somatic order in which we live and that lives in us. These "experiences," notes Fine (1995:256), "provide the basis for comparative judgment" and evaluation. Reflexive rituals are the somatic and symbolic material we employ in typifications of the self such as personal, social, and situational identities. Somatic rituals are habits of sensing and sense-making which are intimately linked to one another, and thus to a sense of self, as they "reach deep into our personal lives, all day, every day" (Synnott 1993:187). When considered as a whole, these rituals comprise the self's *somatic career*: a living history of the sensuous self and its orientation to future somatic work.

In order to understand and unpack the dynamics of the sensuous self, it is necessary to understand the significance of ritual sensations. In Chapter 3 we focused on the performative dimension of sensations-as-ritual—and quite appropriately, as all rituals are dramas and all dramas are performances. But there is more. As patterns of behaviors regularly performed, rituals are activities *to* which and *from* which we assign, fashion, incorporate and shape meaning over time, out of which selfhood emerges. We can distinguish between two types of sensuous rituals: *ritual sensations* and *sense-making rituals*.

Ritual Sensations and Sense-making Rituals

Ritual sensations are habits. A habit is not to be confused with a blind way of falling into a groove (see Crossley 2001; Dewey 1934). It is a learned sense-making pattern cemented by layers of individual biography and collective memories (Dewey 1934). A habit is an embodied tool for the expression and articulation of perspective and selective attention (Csordas 1993). In Mead's (1938:7) words, a habit tunes an individual or a group into a way of paying attention "which answers both to [the perceiver's] immediate sensitivities and to his [or her] experience." Ritual sensations thus involve both "an immediate sensuous stimulation and an attitude toward this stimulation, which is that of the reaction of the individual to the stimulation" (Mead 1938:3). Such attitude is ritualized because we take it from past experience and re-enact it. We acquire it as a performative skill, and root it in bodily craft. Ritual sensations are thus not to be confused with mechanical sensory responses to material stimuli, but are rather body techniques that guide the material of perception, much like a filtering mechanism.

Cohen's (2006) analysis of the significance of smells in Bangkok provides a useful example of this filter and its role in evaluating the qualities of sensation. According to him, the fact that Thais take great care in detecting bodily odors and in assigning positive valence to bodily perfume, while remaining utterly unconcerned with the stench of public streets, reflects a uniquely Thai attitude toward different moral codes of personal and civic cleanliness, and thus illustrates how ritual perception is the result of a habitual "elaboration and interpretation of . . . impressions" (Cohen 2006:127).

On the other hand, *sense-making rituals* refer to expression and invocation. At the individual level, we use sense-making rituals to sense the continuity of self and establish identity. We do so by expressing the meaningfulness of sensations. At the collective level, we use sense-making rituals to affirm and support the social relationships that underlie the bonds among us. We do so by evoking the agreed norms of our cultural "sensory model" (Classen 1990: 722). If ritual sensations refer to interpretive perception, sense-making rituals refer to public drama and storytelling—cultural and social performance (Turner and Schechner 1988). Through sense-making rituals, individuals and groups "align" (Stokes and Hewitt 1976) conduct with the dominant somatic order of a society. Sense-making rituals may be private and idiosyncratic or openly public, shared, and embodied in formal cultural performances. However, regardless of the social domain in which they take place, they result in materializing (Gell 2006) sensations and in reproducing the means utilized by a society to regulate the senses.

Among the most obvious and ordinary examples of sense-making rituals are our daily social performances of personal odorizing and deodorizing, our mundane practices of odor attraction and avoidance (see Largey and Watson 1972), and our evaluative judgment and categorization of smells (see Low 2005). More formalized cultural performances include the ritual burning of incense associated with many religious ceremonies (Largey and Watson 1972), bathing to purify one of the presence of evil, or any of the other rituals discussed by Howes (1987) or Classen, Howes, and Synnott (1993).

Kelvin Low, in particular, offers an interesting, if not amusing, illustration of the significance of the sensuous self. Sensations are the basis of the embodied self. And, as Low (2005:405) has argued, smell (in particular) "functions as a social medium employed by social actors towards formulating constructions/judgments of race-d, class-ed and gender-ed others, operating on polemic/categorical constructions (and also, other nuances between polarities) which may involve a process of *othering*" in which "an individual defines the self through a difference in smell, and also negates the other as the not-I based on a difference in odours." One of the ways in which Low explored these dynamics was through olfactory breaching experiments in which he violated taken-for-granted norms so he could watch and see how people repair or reconstruct the breach.

Together, ritual sensations and sense-making rituals situate the self within a particular place and time. Particular sensations—for example, those associated with specific toys, nature sounds, music, foods, beverages, even medicinal treatments such as Vaporub®—can serve as nostalgic reminders of past times, places, people, and events (Hirsch 2006). Of all the senses, olfaction is especially capable of evoking the past (Engen 1991; Proust 2001; Schab and

Crowder 1995). Natural scientists reduce this phenomenon by inciting the direct connection of smell to the limbic region of the brain—the region where memories and emotions are stored (Gilbert 1995). Apparently, signals from other senses have an indirect route to this part of the brain, thus resulting in a less powerful association. These physiological mechanisms aside, as we will soon illustrate, strong nostalgic associations are also emergent in both socialization to olfactory sensations (Herz 2006) and active meaning-making processes as individuals "emplace" particular smells and, in the process, perform selfhood. As we will see, these emergent acts of sense-making consist of somatic work that facilitates self continuity over time. As Low (2005:398) succinctly puts it, "smell may be utilized as a social medium in the (re)construction of social realities," and such processes magnify the role of sensations in producing sociality and identity, as well as reproducing a sensory order and culture (Classen 1990; Howes 1991, 2003, 2005; Rodaway 1994; Simmel 1997). Let us then take a look at how recollection creates a *sense* (literally) of self.

THE FORMATION OF SENSUOUS SELFHOOD AND IDENTITY THROUGH RECALLING AND REMEMBERING

As we explained above, selfhood is not an object that pre-exists a person. Rather, selfhood—just like identity—is a process and a product. The senses are crucial in establishing selfhood and identity. Through the senses and sensations we can establish feelings of attachment and unity, and at times even contest the sensory orders that structure our experiences and constrain our actions, affiliations, and preferences. Take eating. The consumption of food and the appreciation of that food's aromas can do much more than fill the stomach. For example, as Law (2001) explains, for Filipino domestic workers employed in Hong Kong, the consumption of Filipino food and the appreciation of its unique smells can carve a meaningful symbolic space in an otherwise foreign and often hostile environment. Cooking, eating, and smelling Filipino food articulate a meaningful Diasporic identity through which Filipino workers dislocate the authoritative spaces of Hong Kong and affirm the existence of a collective identity abroad. In doing so, Filipino women also redefine their own subjectivity. No longer mere "maids," by sharing food's tastes and aromas they recall and re-establish their memories of home and their sense of self:

> Ask any Filipino domestic worker what they do in Hong Kong on a Sunday, and you will be told about the spectacular gathering dubbed "Little Manila." In and around Central Hong Kong more than 100,000 Filipino women cast off the cultural conventions of their Chinese employers for one day a week, and eat Filipino food, read Filipino newspapers/magazines and consume products from an abundant number of Filipino speciality shops . . . One Sunday I entered the park, and rather than being surrounded by

great gatherings of Filipino women was overwhelmed by that marvellous aroma of Indonesian clove cigarettes. Wandering around Victoria Park, for me at least, confirmed statistics of the growing number of Indonesian domestic workers in Hong Kong. Although women from the Philippines have dominated this labour market since the 1970s, there were 31,800 domestic workers from Indonesia in 1998. In Victoria Park they too were enjoying their day off. The fact that the aroma of cloves and chatter in Indonesian dialects could elude Yang, or indeed that signs prohibiting hawking and littering had been posted in Tagalog and not Bahasa Indonesia, merely demonstrates the powerful associations between "Filipino" and "domestic worker" in Hong Kong.

(Law 2001:265–266)

Of course, selfhood is formed in many different ways, through many different processes, and it is impossible to examine all of these—if an exhaustive list could even be compiled. Therefore, aiming for depth rather breadth seems like a logical course of action for the remainder of this chapter. We begin by examining the formation of selfhood in the context of recollection. By recalling and remembering, we shape a sense of self that is deeply unique to each of us, yet common memories are also at the basis of collective identities. After discussing the dynamics of recollection, we shift our emphasis to the presentation of self. We routinely express aspects of ourselves by communicating information to others, and much of this information is of a sensory nature. Our data allow us to examine in particular what we convey about ourselves to others through the way we smell. But we begin with the aromas of recollection.

As Synnott (1991:438) has argued, "odours define the individual and the group." Indeed, as we found in our study of olfaction and nostalgia (Waskul, Vannini, and Wilson 2009), when asked about their "favorite smell," about 70 percent of our respondents include aspects of their individual biographic past and memories of significant others. In most instances, our informants favor particular smells because they connect them to particular people and places about which they are nostalgic. For example, Melissa (age twenty-eight) identifies fresh, clean laundry as her favorite smell because it reminds her of "hanging out with my aunt in England. I used to stay with her for weeks when I was there and she was always doing laundry." For Cindy (age thirty-six), Alberta wild roses remind her "of my grandmother and of when I was a child visiting her home." Frank (age forty-five) associates the smell of lavender with "family, home, and safety," as he recalls his maternal grandmother's room always smelling of the herb. Allison (age thirty-two) writes:

My favorite smell is an unusual one but it is truly the best smell I can think of. It is the smell of my own skin but only in a particular circumstance. Many things need to happen first in order for the smell to occur. The smell occurs only in the summer on a particular[ly] warm day after time spent

> outside, usually at the lake or beach and after remnants of sunscreen, salt, new sweat, grass, and fresh water have melded into one distinct odor on my skin at the end of the day. I think that I am particularly fond of this smell because it happens so rarely now but reminds me of days gone by when, as a child, I had months of opportunities to smell this odor. It represents happy fun filled summers that seemed to go on for ever, holidays spent at my grandparents' home on Gabriola Island [British Columbia, Canada], and fun with friends at the local lakes. It is the one scent that makes me believe if I close my eyes that I am a child again.

Allison's complex and vivid description of olfactory perception not only conveys somatic experiences but shows that those are mediated by memory and nostalgia. As we will soon see, her description also illustrates how embodied identity works. In her own words, Allison astutely describes a fundamental pragmatic relationship: the meaning of memory, sensory perception, and nostalgia do not exist prior to experience, but flow from it in active ritual sensations and sense-making rituals. Let us examine these interrelated processes more closely.

Dewey (1967:154) defines memory as "knowledge of particular things or events once present, but no longer so." Equally, as Allison remarks in the quote above, she is fond of the smell she describes because it "reminds me of days gone by when, as a child, I had months of opportunities to smell this odor." These sentiments are easy to understand and not particularly surprising. However, what needs emphasizing is that these memories are no mere static reservoir of things or events that occurred in the past. Instead, Allison produces these perceptions and memories by active "idealizing activity." It is to this type of idealizing activity that we refer when we use the concept of sense-making ritual. A sense-making ritual—as with any ritual—performs a reality into being and allows it to be sensible. As Dewey (1967:155) explains:

> the object of memory does not exist as a *thing* in space, but only as a mental image. The table which I perceive is one really there in space. The table which I remember exists only in the form of an image in my mind. The perceived table is solid and resists. The remembered table has no physical properties of this kind. The memory of the color red is not itself red, nor is the memory of the odor of a rose fragrant . . . the experiences with which memory deals are, *per se*, wholly ideal. They exist only as results of the constructive activity of intelligence.

Allison's remarks in the previous extract articulate this idealizing activity well; she describes the odor as representing "happy fun filled summers that seemed to go on forever, holidays spent at my grandparents' home on Gabriola Island, and fun with friends at the local lakes." These elements of somatic perception are not denotative of the odor itself and its immediate source but *connotative*.

In other words, they are evaluative, but only in the context of Allison's unique biography. This sense-making practice is distinctive to Allison and only possible by her idealizing and performative activity. These memories are thus not passive records but *acts* Allison produces to shape her sense of bodily self, and ground it into sensations she experienced and revisits. For these reasons, as a product of idealizing activities, memories are "versatile, resourceful interpretive models and cultural schemes" (Rapoport, Lomsky-Feder, and Heider 2002:176).

Many of our participants similarly develop their memory as a connotative and performative activity that significantly intersects with ritual sensations of unique "smellscapes" (Porteous 2006:91):

> One of the most pleasurable odors I recall is from my childhood—it was during the fall in Edmonton when my parents would make mustard pickle[s]. This would take an entire weekend and involved the chopping and cutting of cauliflower, peppers, onions, etc. and the very strong scent of vinegar and mustard would take over our house. It was a happy memory of my parents together in the kitchen, engaging in a ritualistic activity as the coziness of fall and autumn surrounded us.
>
> (Rose, age thirty-nine)

> One of my favorite smells is that of fresh baked bread. It reminds me of many things including my grandmother, my mother, my brother and I making numerous loaves to get ready for winter in Alberta. It has associated with it thoughts of a warm kitchen, important people in my life and the taste of fresh bread still hot from the oven with melted salty butter on it.
>
> (Frank)

As these quotes suggest, the idealizing activity of olfactory perception is often associated with specific scents (and tastes as well, of course). While Rose and Frank focus on the aromas of mustard pickles and freshly baked bread as key to their ritual sensations, others' idealizing activities so resonate with olfactory perception that specific odors are absorbed by the ritual activity, not an odor *per se*. In other words, specific odors are utterly rapt by vivid memories (on this phenomenon, also see Gell 2006). Consider, for example, Amy's (age thirty-one) pleasure in the odor of "baking." She does not identify precise aromas but ties her olfactory perception to memories of performing ritual activities and the feelings she associates with them:

> The most pleasurable odor I can recall is baking. I associate this odor with yummy treats, my family, holidays, or celebrations. My mother always baked a lot at Christmas. I don't bake a lot now—mostly for special occasions and baking always makes me think of something special. The

smell of baking makes me think of a cozy house on a cold night with my family sitting around with a treat after dinner.

Amy merges her fondness for the odor (and taste, too) of "baking" with a ritual practice, but baking does produce scents that she is perhaps unable to convey specifically, owing to the paucity of language to describe odor (Synnott 1993). However, other participants approach this social performance of "routine" (Almagor 1990:257) and ritual (Turner and Schechner 1988) as so central that, ironically, the physiological apperception of odor itself is apparently neither significant nor directly related to the reported olfactory perception. In these cases the connotative elements of olfactory perception completely engulf the reported somatic experience; the perception of odor *is* the ritual feeling that they evoke. In other words, ritual sensations and sense-making rituals are often so intertwined that it is impossible to disentangle them. This is the mark of a true dialectical process: *making sense of a sensation creates a feeling*. Similarly, we make sense of a sensation by relying on ritual and habit. Just as Mead found the presence of a blind spot in the process of constitution of self—a blind spot that makes it impossible to see the I but not the Me, or the Me but not the I—we find that it is impossible to investigate ritual sensations without taking into consideration sense-making rituals. Consider, for example, Rachel's (age forty-nine) olfactory sense-making ritual: her favorite smell isn't a scent at all, but a synaesthetic feeling that she associates with something that is actually odorless:

> If I have to have one favorite smell, it would have to be "sunshine." When I was thinking of this question, I realized that all of my nominees for favorite are variations on a theme, and they all involve warmth from the sun, all in the natural world, and usually feature [some] sort of wildflower (but not always). In the north, without sunshine there really are no smells . . . One key element that binds all of these instances into one "smell memory" is taking the time to feel the sun, to savor the moment, and reflect on my good fortune to live where I can appreciate the gifts of nature.

These reflections illustrate Dewey's (1967:156) insight that both memory and perception are "active construction[s] by the mind of certain data." That is, "we perceive only by bringing past experiences to bear upon the present, so as to interpret it" (1967:157). From this perspective, Dewey (1967:157; emphasis added) identifies three principal ways in which memory is linked to perception: "What memory does is (1) simply to disengage some one of these experiences from its absorption in the perception, giving it an independent *ideal existence*; (2) at the same time interpreting it in such a way that it stands for or symbolizes certain *relations of time*; and (3) *gets its place* in the course of experience."

Dewey's thoughts are quite germane to our use of the concept of ritual. A ritual is first and foremost a generative performance (Turner and Schechner

1988). Sense-making rituals consist of *sense acts* (Austin 1962): acts through which we do not just note the previous existence of something, but through which we perform and generate something into existence. And one of the things—arguably the most important—that we generate is our self as a relationship between us and others in time and place. These relationships between memory and olfactory perception appear repeatedly in our data. Take, for example, how memory influences Nathan's (age thirty-two) olfactory sensation, and how—in making sense of it—he performs a unique sense of self grounded in time and place and in relation with others:

> My most pleasurable recent smell memory would have to be the smell of cumin, cloves, nutmeg, sugar, and other spices brewing in a pot of Indian *chai masala* (spiced tea). Not only does this remind me of how wonderful a cup of chai tastes, but it also triggers memories of a recent trip I took to the Indian subcontinent. The smell holds pungent notes of spice, bitterness, and caramelized sugar. Pure heaven! If I close my eyes when I smell that scent I can not only see the thriving street culture, but it also recalls for me the hum of a vibrant people. The image that comes to mind immediately, however, is sipping a fragrant brew while joining in Buddhist morning prayers at a 1300 year old monastery.

Precisely as Dewey suggested, memory plays a key role in Nathan's perception of chai tea. The odor reminds him "of how wonderful a cup of chai tastes" but, more importantly, the *memory* of "a recent trip I took to the Indian subcontinent" prevents immediate somatic absorption. Instead, the sense-making ritual symbolizes those relations in time. As Nathan puts it, "when I smell that scent I can not only see the thriving street culture, but it also recalls for me the hum of a vibrant people." This memory gives Nathan's olfactory perception a place in the course of experience: "sipping a fragrant brew while joining in Buddhist morning prayers at a 1300 year old monastery" is brought to bear on Nathan's perception of the odor.

Aroma and Nostalgia

> Smell is a potent wizard that transports us across thousands of miles and all the years we have lived. The odor of fruits wafts me to my southern home, to my childhood frolics in the peach orchard. Other odors, instantaneous and fleeting cause my heart to dilate joyously or contract with remembered grief.
>
> (Helen Keller, cited in Synnott 1991:441)

Dewey's reflections on the significance of memory to sensuous perception point at the experience of nostalgia. Though originally a diagnosable disease (the word was coined by Swiss physician Johannes Hofer in the late seventeenth century), nostalgia today refers to a bittersweet emotion: a longing for a sense of both a time and a place anchored in the biographical past. From our pragmatist perspective, that which we fondly recall may or may not *really* have been the way we remember it. There is clearly a great deal of selective perception and even fantasy involved in our nostalgic longings and all of memory. As Wernick (1997:211) has suggested, the time longed for "might never have been present at all. This is probably why nostalgia is sometimes used as a mildly contemptuous descriptor for golden age myths of all kinds." Recall is thus a form of making things happen, a performance, and an action (Connerton 1989). Indeed, recollection is a *sense act*. When we feel nostalgic, we actively create an idealized memory in order to assign people, places, and things to their place. Many participants in our study provide equally evocative accounts of this process:

> To this day, lavender is a smell most associated for me with concepts like family, home and safety. My maternal grandmother was 75 and she lived with us when my brothers were 11 and 7. Her room always smelled like lavender as she had scented shelf paper, a bowl of potpourri, and hand crème from Marks and Spencer all scented with delicate lavender.
>
> (Frank)

> Tommy girl [perfume] is one of my most pleasurable odors. I cannot describe it but it is the fond memories of my relationship with my ex girlfriend that this odor evokes. It really makes me feel happy when I smell it.
>
> (Bruce, age thirty)

As Almagor (1990:258) has remarked, odoriferous sensations are particularly noticeable "when one leaves his society for a while and returns to realize, through their absence, that there are some odorants in the air which characterize his culture." Nostalgia—its etymological origin is the will to "return home"—is thus a typical outcome of olfactory sensations. It is a useful lens to understand both how we make sense of olfaction in precise contexts, and how we connect it to our biographical past.

These data excerpts also point out the evaluative and aesthetic components of nostalgia—indeed, it makes Bruce "*feel* happy" to remember. "Aesthetic" here is meant in the original sense of the word remarked by Dewey (1934). Aesthetics is necessarily sensory (also see Bull, Gilroy, Howes, and Kahn 2006). Moreover, Dewey's insights on perception suggest that aesthetics are not purely cognitive but also sensory. Furthermore, "Sensation is the result of the *activity* of the psycho-physical organism, and is produced, not received" (Dewey 1967:43; emphasis in original). Hence, grounding the idea of a sense act and somatic work in Dewey's philosophy seems entirely appropriate. Recall from an earlier quote how Allison actively produces the description of her favorite aroma: "Many things need to happen first in order for the smell to occur. The smell occurs only in the summer on a particular[ly] warm day after time spent outside, usually at the lake or beach and after remnants of sunscreen, salt, new sweat, grass, and fresh water have melded into one distinct odor on my skin at the end of the day." Kate (age twenty-nine) provides another multi-sensory example of how "smells play an important role" in the "process of ordering [one's] world" (Almagor 1990:257):

> I remember a kid's book called *Pat the Bunny* which has different textures for kids to touch: daddy's rough beard (sandpaper), a shiny mirror, etc. At the end, you got to pat the bunny's belly, which was soft cottony fur and has a very unique smell. I bought the book again several years ago when a friend had a baby and found that it still smells the same—a little bit like baby soap or something, but very distinct. It brings me right back to my childhood. I think it's a combination of a nice, clean, fragrance combined with happy childhood memories (I loved that book and remember reading it with unidentifiable but very nice adults) that makes it so special.

As these quotes suggest, sensation "arouses the mind to put forth effort"—what Dewey 1967:44) calls excitation: "As excitation it [sensation] possesses intensity or degrees of vividness, and is allied to feeling." And, as our data excerpts also suggest, that intensity, its vividness, and associated feelings all have an important temporal dimension: "Sensation *indicates the particular factor* in mental products. That is, it always refers the content in connection with which it is experienced to a *this* and a *now*" (Dewey 1967:44; emphasis in original). For this reason, the pragmatic relationship between sensory perception, memory, and nostalgia represents a significant form of identity work and somatic work by bodying forth a past sense of self into a current one, and a current sense of self into earlier sensations. Thus, in the words of Almagor (1990:267; emphasis added), familiar odors will "*transform* a person at once, to a point of time in the past." Similarly, Howes (1987:399) speaks of "transubstantiation."

Transformation, or transubstantiation, is the outcome of commemorative rituals, the sedimentation of past into the body (Connerton 1989:72). A memory is more than a mere text or discourse. By recollecting, we incorporate the past. As Connerton (1989:71) puts it, "what is remembered in commemorative ceremonies is something in addition to a[n] . . . organized variant of personal of cognitive memory." A sense-making ritual is a performance of habituation and the habituation of sensation "in the bodily substrate of the performance" (1989:71). Recall how Allison's ritual sensation of a particular odor makes her "believe if I close my eyes that I am a child again"—a sentiment expressed in nearly identical words by several other participants. In this fashion, particular odors (in this case) can trigger memories that point to other past sensory experiences, or remind us of times, places, or people that evoke special emotions. Thus, we actively employ memory and nostalgia not only in olfactory perception but in embodied identity work that evokes old selves. These old selves reminisce with the present self by virtue of both their differences (places, people, and circumstances that are no longer present) and their similarities (namely, they were experienced by the same embodied person). Put differently, in recalling, I reflect on past experiences—"I" experienced those ritual sensations and through ritual recollections the "me" can make sense of my self-anchoring in time (Mead 1934). In this way, *recalling is a form of somatic work: a sensual practice we actively deploy to maintain self continuity over time.* Consistent with Mead (1929), the present attends to what we recall and the past aids to structure the present (Rapoport, Lomsky-Feder, and Heider 2002; Schwartz 1991; Schwartz, Zerubavel, and Barnett 1996). The following quote captures these dynamics beautifully:

> When I was a child, I noticed that the air smells very sweet and clean right after a rainstorm. It usually happens just after the rain has finished falling, when there's still some dampness in the air. That's my favorite smell. It's so clean and inviting. The smell brings back memories of spending my childhood summers, camping on Vancouver Island. It frequently rained and that's exactly the way it smelled. Every time I smell that aroma now, it reminds me of all the fun times we had as a family.
>
> (Leah, age twenty-nine)

If thinking is, as Mead (1934) would have it, an internalized conversation, then memories are a special form of talking to oneself. What is memory if not a highly specialized form of self dialogue? Only here, unlike Mead's framework, the dialogue is neither bound to language nor role-taking *per se* (both of which are arguably overemphasized in Meadian pragmatism and the Mead–Blumer thread of symbolic interactionism). Language plays a limited role because recalling is an act that is overwhelmingly *sensory* and loaded with potent *emotional* capital (individually or collectively). Recalling, in the words of Connerton (1989:22), has "the capacity to reproduce a certain performance." That is, recalling is a ritual practice that generates the past in richly vivid and sensory ways, and these serve to ground expressive self continuity over time and in place. Through sense acts, such as recollections, the sensuous self connects odors to people, places, activities, or feelings. In the words of Serematakis (1994:37), recalling is a form of sensuous commensality, an "exchange of sensory memories and emotions and of substances and objects incarnating remembrance and feeling." This can be seen in the following extract:

> My Dad was a logger and lived in a camp all week . . . Fridays were a much anticipated highlight of the week, because that meant that Dad was coming home. We'd watch from the window to see his car coming down the road, and then he would be there. My brother and I would jostle for

> the honor of carrying his suitcase or lunch bucket from the car. And when the suitcase was opened (there was often the chance that chocolate bars would be found) the kitchen would fill with the smell of wool and sawdust and sweat and chainsaw oil: Dad. A whiff of that combination today sends me back to being a little girl and giving my Dad a welcome home hug.
>
> (Rachel)

These data provide support for Davis's assertion that nostalgia facilitates the continuity of identity. In his words (Davis 1979:31), nostalgia possesses a "powerful benchmarking potential"; that is, nostalgia enables one to "locate in memory an earlier version of self with which to measure . . . some current condition of the self." Previous studies have looked at such phenomena as "displaced nostalgia" (that is, individuals expressing nostalgia for times not known to them first-hand), the important function that reminiscing can play among those suffering from dementia (for example, the practice of Reminiscence Therapy), and the role of objects in maintaining identity. Olfaction plays a vital role in one's active (re)construction of the past, and in establishing a somatic sense of self through time—that is, nostalgically "connecting" (Lankauskas 2006:40) then and "now" and thereby linking "former sensuous self" and "present sensuous self." We employ a number of strategies as we attempt to maintain a stable self over time, and active reminiscing is one of them. Reminiscences and nostalgia may seamlessly flow from the "placing" of a specific aroma; that is, from the incorporation of memory into flesh and self (Connerton 1989). We are not saying, "You are what you smell," but we are saying that those experiences we associate with particular smells can be highly relevant to the processes of sensuous self construction, (re)construction, and self identity.

THE PRESENTATION OF THE SENSUOUS SELF

"That which we call a rose by any other word would smell as sweet." So muses Juliet in Shakespeare's famous tragedy (Romeo and Juliet, Act II, Scene 2). Notwithstanding romance—in fact, quite to the contrary—sensory perception in general, and olfactory perception in particular, is not so simple. Sensory perception hinges on active sense-making. For example, as we have illustrated, we make odor meaningful through active reminiscing, formulating chains of associations, evaluating and interpreting the significance of unique biographical particulars, the social norms of olfactory communities, and the indexical properties and qualities of odors themselves. Through smell, we reflexively assign meaning unto odor and, for this reason, odor is also a "sign vehicle" (Goffman 1959): we manipulate and manage it on our bodies and in our environments to convey desired impressions. For example, as Peter (age fifty-seven) suggests, "There is a manipulative element to controlling odors." Indeed, odor conveys meaning and is therefore a significant element of the dramaturgies of everyday life. As we illustrate below, we often manage our olfactory impression in positive and negative interpersonal rituals, reward people who perform those well, and stigmatize those who violate them.

Goffman (1967:45) points out that "the general capacity to be bound by moral rules may well belong to the individual, but the particular set of rules which transforms him into a human being derives from requirements established in the ritual organization of social encounters." Likewise, constructions of odor, olfactory somatic rules, and perceptions of smell permeate the normative dramaturgies of everyday life. We rely on them to present our selves and to reward or reject others. In this way "the physical and the moral are united in odour" (Synnott 1993:191) and represent a genuine form of somatic surveillance, as evidenced by Nichole (age forty), who wrote, "Personal body odor is something that I prefer to keep under control at all times, regardless of whether I am in public or not."

For these reasons, people are often "dramaturgically aware" (Brissett and Edgley 1990) of the significance of odor in impression management—and particularly in terms of the implications for "face" (Goffman 1967:5)—"the positive social value a person effectively claims . . . in terms of approved social attributes." According to Synnott (1993:187), "smelling good is a sign of being good." Rose confirms this: "Just like looks smell is tied to impression; if you want to make a good one you need to smell nice." Likewise, Steve (age fifty-six) writes, "I think you can lose credibility with people if odor is not controlled." This is a sentiment that is widely shared: "Anytime I expect to be in close proximity to others, like at a Doctor's appointment or church, are times that I pay particular attention to how I smell" (Allison); "It is important for me to smell good when I am with other people. It makes me feel good about myself and then I can focus on other people rather than worrying about the impression that I am making" (Chandra, fifty-three).

Goffman (1967:10) suggested that "just as the member of any group is expected to have self-respect, so also [she/]he is expected to sustain a standard of considerateness," an idea that applies to odors. Because odor conveys meaning, it both reflects character and expresses to others an awareness of and commitment to olfactory rules of decorum. Allison expresses this well: "smelling good gives the impression that I take care of myself and have consideration for others who have to spend time with me."

It would seem that olfactory impression management is imperative, especially in situations that we deem important. In these situations we see most clearly the kind of olfactory somatic work we perform "to counteract 'incidents'—that is, events whose effective symbolic implications threaten face" (Goffman 1967:12). In these situations, we routinely engage in *positive* interpersonal rituals (Goffman 1971:63)—those rituals that "affirm and support the social relationship" between odors and their source. For example,

Amy explains why she was especially motivated to smell pleasant on her wedding day:

> I was very conscious of wanting to smell good on my wedding day. Like every bride, I wanted to look beautiful and was afraid that I would get hot and sweaty in my big, heavy dress on a hot August day. I was aware that I would be hugged and kissed a lot on that day and that I would be talking to a lot of people (most of my closest family and friends, in fact) and for that reason was wanting to smell good.

Romantic encounters—or circumstances where romance is possible—are also commonly cited as important moments for acute olfactory dramaturgical awareness and positive interpersonal olfactory ritual:

> The greater the chance of intimacy the more important smelling good is. Walking the dog Saturday morning—don't care about my smell. Going to work—clean and fresh is good enough, no reason to break out the Baldessarini. Dancing, or any social situation where one is likely to get close to women, one wants to avoid being repugnant.
>
> (Peter)

"I like to smell good by applying perfume when I go out with my husband on a rare dinner date or to the movies" (Allison).

In addition to personal odor, we are dramaturgically aware of the significance of environmental olfactory impression management. In our research, informants commonly expressed concern about managing odor in the *places* they inhabit. Ashley (age forty-eight) explained that the smell of a home reflects on its residents, and others express similar sentiments. As Jenna (age thirty-three) writes:

> A home must have controlled smells. No one wants to be in a home with offensive or too strong smells. No one would visit a smelly home and the occupants might carry the smells outside of the home with them making them unpleasant to be around (i.e. mold, cigarette smoke, crazy strong perfume).

Our participants also identified work environments as important places for the management of odor, and not only in terms of the previously mentioned olfactory political correctness. Thus, it is not surprising that Susan (age twenty-five) is especially aware of her olfactory impression management during important work-related meetings and interactions with clients:

> It is particularly important for me to smell good when I am meeting clients—especially for the first time. Smell is such an important part of a

person, whether you realize it or not, that a bad odour can break what could have been a great relationship! Before a meeting, I usually eat a mint, and wash my hands so I can be sure that I am presenting myself in the best way possible. Also, wearing clean clothes, bathing, and not going out the night before helps too! . . . I don't want to be remembered by a stench!

Restaurants were also identified as important environments for the control of odor. Kate claims that "food is so tied with smells," while Melissa writes:

> Smell definitely impacts the sense of taste. The sense of smell is being used to its fullest in a restaurant with all the culinary smells about . . . Good smells seem to enhance taste, and bad smells can just ruin the whole experience. Food establishments control smell also by putting familiar smells out to the public: popcorn at movies, fries from McDonald's (I've heard they fan it into the air outside). Smell is very important to sales I would imagine.

Informants commonly cited bathrooms as among the most important environments for the control and manipulation of odor. Just as the smell of flatulence, urine, and feces contaminates the offender's moral and aesthetic character, it can pollute an entire environment. As Cahill (1985:43) explains, "because the profaning power of odor operates over a distance and in all directions, moreover, individuals who defecate in . . . bathrooms not only temporarily profane themselves but also risk profaning the entire setting." However, because bathrooms are *the* designated place for "creature releases" (Goffman 1963:69)—and all creatures must release—they are also social environments rife with *negative* interpersonal rituals (Goffman 1971:62) that involve honoring the "individual's right to private 'preserves' and 'to be let alone'" (Cahill 1985:39). But adherence to this negative interpersonal ritual—especially in private bathrooms—entails a "dual set of issues for the offender and the offended" (Goffman 1971:100). On the one hand, those who encounter the smells that emulate from a bathroom must dutifully honor the negative ritual through "tactful blindness" (Goffman 1955:219). On the other hand, those who produce the smell are "responsible for trying to make amends for his [or her] offense *and* for showing proper regard for the process of correction" (Goffman 1971:100; emphasis in original). Therefore, as Nichole suggests: "Like many people, I feel the need to remedy bathroom odors when they occur. Although everybody experiences and contributes to these odors, it seems important to hide them when they happen."

"In our society, defecation involves an individual in activity which is defined as inconsistent with the cleanliness and purity standards expressed in many of our performances," writes Goffman (1959:121), and even its smell is a possible expressive and impressive hazard. Indeed, failure to control the odors of flatulence, feces, and urine in the bathroom is a potential dramaturgical catastrophe—a source of looming prospective embarrassment, regardless of whether the bathroom is in a home or a work environment, for public or private use:

> [It is important to control odor in t]he bathroom: because it is a publicly used space and is often associated with negative smells resulting from bodily elimination. I leave a box of matches in the bathroom for guests or family members to light after using the toilet. I find the smell of burnt sulphur more appealing than artificial sprays. If odor is not controlled in these places then it may leave a bad impression for guests who visit our home. It is almost as if when a person uses the bathroom they want to feel as if they were the first and only one to use it. It is unpleasant to be reminded that anyone visited the space before them.
>
> (Allison)

In conclusion, as we have seen in great detail throughout this chapter, the senses are critical to the development and expression of selfhood and identity. Not only do we routinely derive a sense of self by establishing what we like and dislike; we categorize others on the basis of whether and why we like or dislike them. These basic expressions of liking articulate our feelings, and feelings are often other words for sensations. In sum, the senses and sensations are crucial media for the constitution of subjectivity and for how we relate to one another.

6

A SENSE OF PLACE, A SENSE OF TIME

The forming of the five senses is a labor of the entire history of the world down to the present.

(Marx 1967:46)

One of the central claims of Zionism was that the Jews lived a disembodied existence in exile and that only a healthy national life could restore a necessary measure of physicality or materiality. Zionism meant not only the physical rooting of "people of the air" . . . in the soil of Palestine, but the reclamation of the body.

(Biale 1992:283)

"*Baruch Ha ba le Israel.* Welcome to Israel," says the gorgeous, smiling soldier at the immigration desk of Tel Aviv's Ben Gurion Airport. "Can I see your Israeli identity card?" she asks, examining my (Simon's) Belgian passport and my US Green Card.

"Israeli identity card? I don't have it," I respond, a bit confused.

Frowning impatiently, she looks at her computer screen and asks: "Didn't you used to live in Israel?"

I chuckle, amazed that their computer records still contain this information after nearly thirty years. "Well, yes, you're right," I answer, "I lived in Israel between 1975 and 1983, but I do not have my Israeli identity card." I sense her disapproval. Not because I do not have an Israeli identity card, but because I had decided to leave the country a long time ago, before she was even born.

The Hebrew language describes my status in Israel in terms that clearly suggest physical movement *with* social evaluation (Bar-On 2008): one does not "immigrate" into Israel, one "ascends" or "rises" (*oleh*) to it. Conversely, one does not "emigrate" from Israel, one "descends" (*yored*) from it. By immigrating, we elevate our status; we become and feel taller. By emigrating, we slide down the prestige slope; we become and feel smaller. The valuational charge these words contain becomes even clearer a few days later, at the bank where I exchange my US dollars for Israeli shekels. Like so many Israelis who see my foreign documents, the teller asks me where I learned to speak Hebrew. As usual, I answer that I used to live here. Turning to her colleague, the teller explains: "Tamar, this young man used to live here, but then left us [*azav otanou*]." While her tone sounds like she is taking my departure personally, her choice of the pronoun "us" indicates the collective consequences of my past decision. With its connotations of personal relations, the word *azav* (left, abandoned) feels like a sting.

"Have a nice stay," says the gorgeous Israeli soldier at the airport, loudly stamping my passport, no longer smiling.

FORMING SIGHTS

> Ways of seeing are structured and mediated by cultural forms, and by specific kinds of knowledge, which are in turn informed by the act of seeing itself, in a complex circular process. On the basis of that vision and the interpretation of it, courses of action are chosen by individuals.
>
> (Hockey and Collinson 2007:121)

I will never forget the first time I traveled to Israel. The year was 1968, one year after the Six-Day War. I was eight years old, and my mother had decided to take my brother and me for the summer there. Giddy with excitement, we took the night train from Brussels to Marseille, where we boarded the ship *Theodor Herzl*—appropriately enough, the name of Zionism's founding father. Then we sailed to Haifa, with stopovers in Naples and Cyprus.

Back then, Israel had international rock star status. Pictures of handsome young Israeli soldiers were adorning the front pages of many Western weekly magazines; and stories, jokes, and songs about the country's recent military victory filled the air. While the mainstream American press had been reliably supportive of Israel, even their typically unfriendly counterparts in France had joined the chorus, drawing parallels between the Israeli Defense Forces' smashing victory over Arab countries and King David's army smiting the Philistines.

Around that same time, with a group of friends, I attended a screening of Otto Preminger's *Exodus* at the Brussels Jewish Community Center. We were mesmerized. Paul Newman's portrayal of Ari Ben Canaan—the youthful, athletic, and heroic Israeli male—was irresistible, especially to young Belgian Jews growing up in the aftermath of the Holocaust and its visual representations. Although these have changed noticeably over the last few decades (see Bar-On 2008; Hazan 2001), in those years they offered very few heroic role models for children like us to emulate. The power of this movie to inflame our imaginations was also boosted by another text. High up on the wall of the auditorium where the movie was screened, a large black-and-white picture of an Israeli man and woman seemed to confirm the factual existence of the mythical Ari Ben Canaan and his female counterpart. Bereft of any text, the picture echoed the main lessons of the movie. Young, attractive, tanned, smiling, casually dressed, a rifle nonchalantly slung over the shoulder, their bodies radiated health and discipline. Looking straight at the camera, their faces communicated a mixture of friendly benevolence and heroic determination. The message seemed to be: "We mean well but we won't hesitate to defend ourselves. Join us in this epic adventure."

My family's bonds to Israel were strong. Having survived the Holocaust, they considered Israel to be simply miraculous and so much more than a microscopic dot on the world map. It was our homeland and shelter where we could be first-class citizens rather than members of an always threatened minority group. It was a military power that could unleash its devastating wrath against any enemy too evil or stupid to want to repeat Hitler's crimes. It was the ancestral soil providing physical proof of our past, a vast "live" archeological site where we could literally see, hear, smell, touch, and walk through all the places mentioned in our sacred texts. It was a holy ground where we could feel closer to God. It was a psychological space of individual redemption and transformation. It was a political arena where we could at last collectively realize our potential as a nation. It was a daring multicultural experiment where a socialist utopia still seemed possible. It was, in short, the Promised Land.

We had many relatives and friends in Israel. My mother had lived there in the 1950s when she was still single, and my father was working as a diplomat at the Belgian Embassy in Tel Aviv. They were divorced by the late 1960s, although my father had hoped that a return to the homeland would prompt a return of the family structure. The uncompromising love of Israel we absorbed at home was also nurtured in most of our social activities. Embracing the virtues of "muscle Judaism" (Presner 2003), many of us trained at the Maccabi Sports Club.[1] On Saturdays, we went to meetings of a Zionist–socialist youth organization where we played sports and attended lectures on socialism, Israeli politics, culture, and society. We learned Israeli songs and folk dances, adopted Israeli first names, watched pro-Israeli movies, and participated in pro-Israel demonstrations. During the week, we attended a Jewish school where we celebrated Israeli holidays and learned—in addition to the standard curriculum—the Torah, Israeli Hebrew, and Israeli history. We were constantly knocking on doors of community members to collect money for Israel. Money to plant Israeli trees, build Israeli hospitals, develop Israeli towns, feed the Israeli poor, and comfort Israeli orphans.

Over the next seven years, I would return to Israel five times; and when I turned fifteen, I left Belgium for good, joined a kibbutz, and lived in Israel until I was twenty-three.

SENSING ZIONISM

> Each place its own psyche. Each sky its own blue.
>
> (Abram 1997:262)

Zionism is not solely an ideology that promotes geographical migration; it also promotes identity transformation, particular ways of being, and a particular "sensory orientation" (Geurts 2002). While the sensory qualities of Zionism have long been ignored in academic discussions and are typically absent from political debates, they should be acknowledged as they have transformative and generative powers. For good and bad.

A few months ago, visiting my mother (who has now permanently resettled in Israel), I decided to develop this chapter by returning to the places I used to frequent so that I might better *make sense* of this sensory orientation, its sources, and consequences. In contrast to Proust, whose memories were triggered by an unexpected and uncontrolled sensation, I actively sought out those sensations that, in turn, serve as the impulse for self-reflection and sociological analysis. As I hope will become clear throughout this chapter, my seemingly private sensory experiences are instances of a socio-political project that shaped and still shapes legions of citizens and immigrants.

Before I proceed, three caveats are in order. First, the present chapter is a modest attempt to produce a piece of sensuous scholarship—a text *about* the senses, *through* the senses, and *for* the senses. As Abram (1997:265; emphasis in original) explains:

> to make sense is to *enliven the senses*. A story that makes sense is one that stirs the senses from their slumber, one that opens the eyes and the ears to their real surroundings, tuning the tongue to the actual tastes in the air and sending chills of recognition along the surface of the skin. To *make sense* is to release the body from the constraints imposed by outworn ways of speaking, and hence to renew and rejuvenate one's felt awareness of the world. It is to make the senses wake up to where they are.

Following the logic of such texts, this chapter is characterized by indeterminacy, performativity, contingency, and emergence. As a reflexive text, it oscillates between sensations and interpretations, biography and history, the sensual and the ideological. Thus, rather than developing grand theories about the social construction of the senses or Zionism, I invite you, the reader, to accompany me on a short guided sensory tour of Israel. As we smell, taste, listen, touch, walk about, and look around, I will try to "make sense" of those experiences by using the scholarship on the senses and on Zionism.

The second caveat is that the purpose of this chapter is, emphatically, *not* to discuss the Israeli–Palestinian conflict or evaluate Zionism as an ideology or a historico-political project. As a former resident of Israel and activist in the Israeli left, I have some knowledge of the agonizing pains each side inflicts on the other, and I do not wish to elaborate on those here.

The final caveat concerns the situatedness of what follows. From Tripoli to Delhi, from Toronto to Rio, from Milan to Tehran, a multitude of immigrants from widely different backgrounds have had to adjust their sensorium to the Israeli "sensory orientation." How they adjusted was and continues to be shaped by a host of complex and interacting factors. Hence, it goes without saying that my experiences in Israel, my adjustment to the Israeli sensory order, and my "sense-making" efforts have been and continue to be informed by my biography and changing social positions. As Feld and Basso (1996:91) have elegantly stated: "as place is sensed, senses are placed; as places make sense, sense makes place."

SMELLING TRANSITIONS

> The olfactory system is tied directly and intimately to the part of our brain most involved with memory and emotion . . . odor is often the mechanism which triggers off (and leads to) changes in our moods, behavior, and thoughts.
>
> (Almagor 1990:253)

Until a decade or so ago, you knew you had landed in Israel just by the unmistakable and omnipresent sweet smell of Time cigarettes mixed with jet fuel. Back then, it seemed that most people smoked Time—the national cigarette, the almost by-default option for Israeli smokers. Men who could afford it or wanted to show off would nonchalantly display a pack of Marlboro Red or Camel tucked under a rolled-up T-shirt sleeve. Women would fish a pack of Kent or Parliament out of their purses or shirt pockets. If you were a smoker in intellectual leftist circles, then Noblesse (*never* American cigarettes) seemed to be de rigueur. Today, with the new anti-smoking regulations, the airport does not smell like anything at all. You could have landed by mistake at Heathrow, JFK, or LAX, and would not know the difference. What a shame, especially considering the importance of smell.

On the other hand, I tell myself that it might be better to ease gradually into the Israeli smellscape. After all, as Howes (1987:410) points out, olfaction is significantly associated with the experience of transition:

> Interpreting transition as meaning "category change," it has been demonstrated that there is an intrinsic relationship between smell and cognitive

transformation at the logical level (smells are most noticeable at boundaries), the psychological level (given the effect of odors on memory and discursive reason), and at the sociological level (smells synchronize the emotional and physical states of the members of a congregation).

Speeding along the freeway, I open my rental car window to "collect data" and recollect experiences. The ninety-minute drive from the airport to Haifa is indeed a succession of curious blends that announce the various cities, settlements, and industrial zones along the way. Benzene and bananas, fertilizers and flowers, sulfur and sea breeze.

It is late when I reach Haifa, but I am wide awake, all my senses alert. As Amit-Kokhavi (2006:143) notes, Haifa's very topography is rich with social and historical significance. Here, "one has to gradually climb up from the shore or port up to the top of the mountain. This in turn creates an up-and-down dichotomy according to which the further up one lives, the higher one's socio-economic status." A second dichotomy, topographically almost identical to the first, represents time: "the binary opposition between (Arab) past and (Jewish) present" (Amit-Kokhavi 2006:144). Although the situation is slowly changing, Haifa's Arabs tend to live mostly in the lower level of the city—slightly above the port, close to the Hadar district. This district is populated by older residents, Mizrachim (Jews of Middle Eastern origins) and orthodox Ashkenazim (Jews of European origins). The top of Mount Carmel is more affluent and offers more green spaces, beautiful vistas, luxurious hotels, expensive boutiques, lavish houses, chic restaurants, and a distinctly Western feel and population. The apex of Mount Carmel—the Denyah district—is the most expensive one; it also houses Haifa University and the prestigious Technion Technological Institute. Each district has its own sounds, smells, rhythms, linguistic inflections, modes of interaction, risks, and opportunities.

I easily find my way to the busy Moriah Boulevard, my old stomping ground. It is a wide commercial avenue that stretches almost in a straight line across the top of Mount Carmel. I park on a small adjacent street and decide to walk around to tune my body up (Goffman 1989) to this once-familiar place. After a while, I choose a café. The lights are soft and the din of conversation is pleasant. I settle by a window overlooking the boulevard, and order. Waiting for the waiter, I close my eyes, open my nostrils, and inhale deeply. The warm smell of baking bread blends with the perfume of cardamom-laced Arabic coffee, the sweet scent of cinnamon on glazed pastry, and the minty steam slowly rising from glasses of hot tea. But my stomach starts to growl, reminding me that I have not eaten in about nine hours. After fifteen minutes or so, I pay my bill and decide to look for food.

I dismiss outright a McDonald's, a Pizza Hut, and other franchises that announce the Americanization of Israeli taste (Azaryahu 2000). Instead, I program my internal GPS to find those aromas that so overwhelmed me the first time I came; those aromas that confirm that this is indeed the Middle

East—a different sensorium and a different mindset. I am searching for those odors that, as Almagor (1990:258) points out, "are noticed and become culturally meaningful when one leaves his society for a while and returns to realize, through their absence, that there are some odorants in the air which characterize his culture. Such smells belong to the whole region or locality, not to individual objects. It is 'the smell of homeland.'"

Walking along Moriah Boulevard, I synchronize my pace and course to the various aromas I encounter along the way. I circle around a dozen small food stands where falafel balls are frying in large oil vats, and juicy sides of lamb sizzle as they slowly rotate in front of fiery red electric grills. I cross over the boulevard and slow down by nearby shops where the smoky fragrance of roasting pine nuts, pistachios, and sesame seeds mingle with ears of corn steaming in deep aluminum drums. A few yards further, I stop by the open door of a spices store and linger for a while in a fragrant bouquet of turmeric, cumin, curry, saffron, and *za'atar*.[2] This little walk does the trick. I feel a bit more grounded, a bit more attuned to the here and now, and, paradoxically, transported back to this same place thirty years ago. But my stomach is still growling.

TASTING IDENTITY

> Information about food must be gathered wherever it can be found: by direct observations in the economy, in techniques, usages, and advertising; and by indirect observation in the mental life of a given society.
>
> (Barthes 1997:20)

Eating, this most necessary physiological function, is shaped by dynamic political, social, cultural, and economic forces. These inform our psychological dispositions toward eating, and everyday practices revolving around it. As Fischler (1988:275) notes:

> Food is central to our sense of identity. The way any given human group eats helps assert its diversity, hierarchy and organization, and at the same time, both its oneness and the otherness of whoever eats differently. Food is also central to individual identity, in that any given human individual is constructed, biologically, psychologically, and socially by the food he/she chooses to incorporate.

What, how, when, why, where, and with whom we eat—or will not eat—shape our engagement with the world, others, and the self (see also Beardsworth and Keil 1997). However, while a scholarship about food is quickly growing in the social and other sciences, it seems that, with rare exceptions (e.g. Choo 2004; Classen 1999; Stoller 1984, 1989), few authors prepare or eat the food they describe in their writings. And while the many ideas produced by this scholarship are doubtlessly interesting and important, in much of this work food seems to remain an object of intellectual dissection rather than of sensory engagement, and it is served accordingly. Since eating is necessary for thinking, a more appetizing sociological treatment of food should blend analysis with sensory attention to—among other topics—its ingredients, the work involved in producing it, the complex social practices surrounding its consumption, and, of course, its taste. After all, according to the local religious texts, knowing-through-eating is the first tragic and defining human act. On a more personal level, Choo (2004:209) also points out that:

> Sensory experiences of food contain memories, feelings, histories, places and moments in time. Likewise, changes in these sensory experiences encode broader societal changes and provide reference points between then and now, here and there. They contain collective embodied memories, encoded by shared experience and points of identification and there is a symbiotic relationship between senses and memory, with sensory experiences contained within memories and at the same time memories contained within sensory experiences, a tantalising co-dependency.

Standing in line at a street falafel stand, I remember how the tastes of Israel awakened me from a deep gustatory slumber the first time I came. The exotic herbs and intoxicating spices, the sweet tropical fruits and spicy condiments, the new shapes, textures, colors, and combinations of Middle Eastern food demanded a conscious readjustment of both taste buds and digestive tract. As I watch customers eating their falafel at the counter, I also remember that the very act of eating here requires a different kind of tactile engagement, as the European etiquette I grew up with has little traction. People use their hands to tear pita pockets in two and to keep the salads, pickled vegetables, and falafel balls from falling out. With large spoons that change hands faster than you can see, they douse the top layer of the pita pocket with thick, creamy *tchina* (tahini) dressing. They are more careful with the *'amba*—that tangy, deep yellow mango curry sauce brought by Iraqi immigrants in the 1950s. One drop of *'amba* on your fingers, and they'll smell for days. If it falls on your shirt, it will probably never wash out. In contrast to Heide Imai's (2008) encounters with Kyoto street vendors, eating at the falafel food stands seems almost to invite interactions between customers. Standing shoulder to shoulder with complete strangers, we strike up spontaneous conversations—about the food, the weather, and, of course, politics. Following the simple rule of turn-taking, we wait for the other to talk so that we can sink our teeth in the rich pita pocket, oblivious to the juices and dressings dripping through our fingers, forming yellowish drops on shoes and sidewalk.

Intermittently wiping my fingers with the rough paper napkins, I remember a scene from my first visit to Israel. Still unschooled in cultural relativism, I had innocently asked Adel—a Druze friend of the family who was hosting a lavish dinner in our honor—about the missing knives and forks on the dinner table. Diplomatically ignoring my relatives' obvious embarrassment caused by my tactless question, Adel laughed. "Forks? Knives? I don't know where they've been." Extending his right hand, he then added, "These fingers, I know *exactly* where they've been." Forsaking years of European cuisine and having access only to locally produced food, it seemed that the project of becoming Israeli included touching my food, licking my fingers, training my tongue to tame the sharp tastes and teaching my lips to embrace the edible fires. It also required disciplining my digestive track to adapt to the spicy food, and instructing my body to sweat it out silently, courageously, and without complaint. Like a native.

Israeli food does not just deliver calories to citizens' bodies but helps attune them to the national project, at the gut level. As Fischler (1988:279) remarks, "to incorporate food is, in both real and imaginary terms, to incorporate all or some of its properties. We become what we eat." This approach to food was not lost on the pioneers of the first immigration waves in the late nineteenth and early twentieth century. As Even-Zohara (1981:172) notes,

> Green olives, olive oil and white cheese . . . acquired a clear semiotic status. The by-now-classical literary description of the Hebrew worker sitting on a wooden box, eating Arabic bread dipped in olive oil, expresses at once three new phenomena: a) he is a worker; b) he is a "true son" of the land; c) he is not eating in a "Jewish" way (he is not sitting at a table and has obviously not fulfilled the religious commandment of washing his hands).

The most popular "special" on the Israeli ideological menu is probably the *sabra* fruit (known in the West as the prickly pear). Sabra also refers to a native-born citizen, and connotes, even in the Diaspora, the essence of Israeliness itself. The Sabra was

> a good-hearted, sociable, strong person who was good-looking, with rough edges but a sweet interior like the fruit of the Sabra, a hero who never cries . . . A son of Israel, he symbolizes Israel's sons and daughters in a nation that is being renewed. He gives his life for his country . . . and Israel commemorates his memory forever as part of the cultural memory that is created over the years.
>
> (Bar-On 2008:60–81)

Paradoxically, because the "essential" Israeli qualities embodied by the Sabra still betray European roots, this symbol became vehemently challenged by immigrants originating in Middle Eastern and Asian countries, and the Arab population.[3]

While "we become what we eat," Fischler (1988:280) proposes other social and symbolic effects of eating:

> not only does the eater incorporate the properties of food, but, symmetrically, it can be said that the absorption of food incorporates the eater into a culinary system and therefore into the group which practices it . . . But this is not all: any culinary system is attached to, or part of, a world view, a cosmology.

Orienting oneself to a group's cosmology is achieved not only by food absorption but by participating in its preparation. As Choo (2004:212) explains, "the very process of the production itself contains embodied memories and allows for embodied cultural transmissions." The practices surrounding food consumption (rather than "absorption") also reproduce social relations. For example, Wiggins (2002) demonstrates the bonding functions of vocalizing gustatory pleasures when eating in the company of others; and—at the other extreme—Baudrillard (1989:15) interprets the large number of people eating alone in the streets of major American cities as symptomatic of a broader social and psychological breakdown.

Back in time at the kibbutz, after a hard day's work in the fields, we sit in a semicircle around a small and smoky kerosene heater—the main source of fuel for both warmth and light "cooking." Following the principle of "rotation" of responsibilities that is so central to the kibbutz way of life and economy, today it's my turn to prepare the afternoon snacks. I toast slices of white bread on the little grill that protects the burner of the heater, wait until smoke rises, and flip them over. After a while, I ask Boaz if they're sufficiently toasted. He winks and nods silently. With a pocket knife, I slice one of the avocados I picked today in two, dexterously pop out the thick brown pit, spread a generous layer of the green flesh on the toast, and sprinkle some salt on it. "*Bon appétit*," I say, handing Boaz his toast. They love French. Dror is next, then Yaron, then Amir, then me. Tomorrow, it will be somebody else's turn to "cook." At night, we sneak into the collective dining hall, pick the locks of the industrial-size steel fridges, and select eggs, bread, and vegetables to prepare modest banquets, to which the armed guards are naturally always invited. We do not perpetrate such mischief because we are hungry. Far from it. And the taste and nutritional value of the food we prepare and consume together do not really matter that much. Rather, those well-coordinated "night missions" serve purely as rituals to celebrate our togetherness and our friendship, to share stories, produce new ones, and provide each other with the psychosocial pleasure—especially precious in this community run on collectivist principles—that we belong. While the bland standard kibbutz fare nourishes the body, the various steps involved in its preparation and consumption reinforce the group, its boundaries, and its core values.

SOUNDING IDEOLOGY

> A cross-cultural study of the metaphoric language of the senses has also revealed that in different cultures the sense of hearing is symbolically related to proper behaviour. "To hear" stands for "to understand," "to act properly," "to obey."
>
> (Panopoulos 2003:641)

> In order to learn a community's language, suggests Merleau-Ponty, it is necessary simply to begin speaking, to enter the language with one's body, to begin to move within it.
>
> (Abram 1997:83)

Energized by the falafel, I decide to continue my walk down narrow streets that lead to breathtaking vistas of Haifa and the surrounding region. This time, I direct my steps toward the soundscape of nightlife. I walk away from the hissing of buses and the random honking of irritated drivers toward the angry meowing of stray cats fighting on top of large aluminum garbage cans. Emerging from front yards and public parks, the rhythmic sounds of crickets and sprinklers seem to set the beat for children's hesitating piano scales escaping from open apartment windows. A few streets down, the eerie yelping of jackals rising from deep in the *wadis*[4] marks the city's boundaries.

Beep. Beep. Beep. Beep. Beeeeeep. Every hour on the dot, you can hear the familiar sequence of four short electronic beeps followed by a long one, announcing the news from Kol Israel (the Voice of Israel)—the national news radio broadcast. In cafés and at bus stops, at the beach and the campus cafeteria, the sound of those five beeps often prompts complete strangers to gather around the one person holding a small transistor radio. Members of these spontaneous audiences cock their ears toward the person who, thanks to (most often) his prized possession, gains the temporary status of bearer of news and, for a brief moment, becomes literally the center of attention. As soon as the news broadcast is over, he is repositioned as a pedestrian, a bus passenger, or a sunbather, and has lost his status as quickly as he gained it. Sometimes when the broadcast is concluded, members of the impromptu audience strike up vociferous conversations about the news. And while this ritual seems unique to the particular bus stop, restaurant, or beach I happen to find myself at, in other parts of the city, in other parts of the country, at this very moment, countless individuals find themselves participating in similar small, spontaneous gatherings that coalesce and disperse hourly, to the timing of the national news broadcast. The electronic beeps preparing citizens for the news function a bit like the tolling of church bells calling the faithful to a service. Except that while the tolling can be easily traced to concrete physical and permanent structures, the beeps are mobile and dispersed. Circulating from individual to individual, emanating from random sources, they distribute authority evenly and, every hour, somewhere, mobilize collective attention, impose silence, and produce feelings of solidarity.

While the sounds produced by the Israeli national radio played a key political role in shaping national identity and culture (Penslar 2003), today, of course, with the silent colonization of iPods and other devices delivering customized acoustic pleasures, pedestrians, bus riders, and beachgoers groove to their own sounds and withdraw into their private sonic cocoons. Thanks also to the constantly growing number of radio stations Israelis can access, the unifying sounds of community have become muted, except in times of imminent danger or national crises (e.g. war, terrorist attacks), celebrations (Independence Day), or commemorations (Holocaust Remembrance Day). For example, critically listening to the folk songs played on national radio on the eve of the controversial 1982 war with Lebanon, Amos Oz (2009:343) — one of Israel's foremost writers—acknowledges their power and questions their broadcasting: "To what tribal codes did those melodies address themselves? What did the tribe want to whisper to itself in the few precious hours that were left before it set out to overrun Lebanon . . .? What emotions were those cloying tunes meant to arouse—or to silence?"

Personal audio devices also seem to weaken the well-established Israeli ritual of collective folk singing—yet another mechanism participants use to bond with others, integrate new immigrants, celebrate the land, remember military victories, honor fallen heroes, and reassert commitment to the Zionist project. As Almog Oz (2000:240) explains:

> The words of the songs, expressing love and longing for the land and national hope, as well as their simple melodies, gave these "homeland songs" the character and role of Zionist religious hymns. They . . . played on the most delicate strings of the Israeli soul and left the heart with a feeling of sweet wistfulness and the sense of a common fate.

Looking for Time cigarettes, I stop at a crowded diner. As I am waiting for the owner to finish his conversation with a patron, I detect the sounds of Middle Eastern music flowing from invisible speakers. With its distinctive instruments, rhythms, scales, and vocal modulations, it resonates perfectly with the diner's food, the patrons' accents, and the cooking smells. In contrast to the often plaintive Yiddish music I heard while growing up, Middle Eastern music sounds more optimistic, sunny, energetic, and joyful. It invites different kinds of bodily response, attention, and emotion. Since national origin and social class are strongly correlated in Israeli society, it is not surprising that, as Nocke (2006:152) notes, "'Israeli Mediterranean music' made its commercial debut in 1974 among the vegetable and household appliance stalls in Tel Aviv's central bus station marketplace."

The association of soundscape, place, and politics is, of course, neither new nor unique to Israel. As research from different disciplines suggests, the use of particular musical styles to establish socio-political position and cultural allegiance has a long history and presents many interesting variations (see Futrell, Simi, and Gottschalk 2006; Weinstein 2000; Willis 1978). For example, as Oosterbaan (2009:81) notes in his study of genres in Rio's favelas: "The different music and sounds audible in the favela embodied an assertive identity politics and the preference for certain music was often indistinguishable from the music's ability to epitomize the socio-political position of the enthusiasts."

The inclusion of Middle Eastern music in the Israeli national soundscape was also the object of a long struggle about whether it could legitimately claim to resonate with the essence of "Israeliness" (Nocke 2006; Pilowsky 1985; Regev 1996). Paradoxically, although Middle Eastern music was condescendingly rejected by the European-bred artistic circles when first broadcast on national radio, these sounds originate from right around here, in this region, this landscape, these colors, this weather (see Nocke 2006).

The struggle about which musical sound should be included in the Israeli acoustic sensory order echoes another dispute about the sounds of nationhood, but this time in the linguistic domain. In the 1920s, well before the establishment of the state, intense rivalries pitted those who demanded that Yiddish become the national language against the "Hebrew Battalions" whose members loudly insisted that only modern Hebrew could articulate the voice of the new nation. As the latter repeated, while Yiddish sounded like Europe, Hebrew announced the Middle East. While Yiddish vocalized the Diasporic Jew, Hebrew declared the birth of the new citizen.

Of course, many immigrants spoke Hebrew in their countries of origin, but there is a significant difference between the Hebrew one stutters in a classroom quiz, murmurs as a prayer, or sings while reading sacred texts, and Hebrew-as-mother-tongue—a language one speaks naturally and fluently to accomplish daily activities in the factory, at the marketplace, on the farm, and on the battlefield. Fortunately, Hebrew won and became, as Helman (2002:359) explains, "a central tool in the invention and consolidation of a new national community. An ideological linguistic hierarchy was created, with Hebrew at the top." Guttural, crisp, strong, informal, and endearingly melodic, modern Hebrew *in its ecological context* was not only a tool for nation-building and citizenship but invited different thoughts, emotions, and ways of being. Eloquently establishing the intimate and powerful relation between ecological context and language, Abram (1997:75; emphasis in original) also notes:

> *We thus learn our native language not mentally but bodily.* We appropriate new words and phrases first through their expressive tonality and texture, through the way they feel in the mouth or roll off the tongue, and it is this direct, felt significance—the *taste* of a word or phrase, the way it influences or modulates the body—that provides the fertile polyvalent source for all the more refined and rarefied meanings which that term may come to have for us.

Of course, it was not sufficient to speak Hebrew fluently. Israeliness also entailed the ability to speak it with the proper accent (Middle Eastern inflections), and—better yet—to insert juicy Arabic idioms nonchalantly into one's delivery.

Street names were also agents of nation-building and acculturation:

> A Zionist writer reported that a *shiver of joy ran through his body* when he first arrived in Tel-Aviv and encountered a Hebrew street sign: "It seems like a small matter, merely street names; but the sweet sound of our own tongue is like a balm for the Jewish soul, after having to hear only foreign sounds all day long."
>
> (Helman 2002:370–371; emphasis added)

Unsurprisingly, changing one's Diasporic name to an Israeli one became, for many immigrants, the most absolute sign of identity transformation, as it publicly declared commitment to the national project in the most personal terms.

The next day, I take my mother for a walk on the beach, and we sit in a small café. From time to time, our conversation is interrupted by the deafening sound of gunfire and the high-pitched mosquito buzz of speedboats. My mother looks a bit anxious. "Nothing to worry about," I tell her. "Navy exercises." The sound of Israeli beaches is punctuated by the unmistakable *pongs* announcing the sport of smash ball. It consists of two players standing across from each other and using large wooden paddles to send a small rubber ball back and forth—without a net. I have rarely seen people playing this sport on American beaches; I have tried to teach it to friends, but found it difficult. Not because my playmates are poor athletes. On the contrary, many play tennis and ping-pong superbly well. What they find difficult to master is resisting the impulse to use the paddle as a launching device that transforms the ball into a dangerous projectile that, they hope, I will fail to catch. Since winning points in tennis or ping-pong requires the other to miss the ball as many times as possible, players necessarily orient to each other and the game itself on the basis of a competitive equation in which "your loss is my gain." By contrast, the object of smash ball is to keep the ball aloft for as long as possible. Following this logic, players must cooperate and adapt the strength, arc, speed, and distance of their exchanges to each other. They will attempt to make it as easy as possible for their counterpart to bounce the ball back their way. Here, the silence of a ball that is not returned is not interpreted as a victory for one player and celebrated with applause. Rather, it is a loss for both sides, and an unfortunate interruption of the game.

Pong . . . . Pong
Pong . . . . . . Pong
Pong . . . Pong
PongPongPongPongPong

The two distinguishable pongs quickly merge into a continuous and accelerating staccato, and the café patrons interrupt their conversation to follow the exchange approvingly. This accelerating sound that blurs the distinction between the two players announces that they are attuned to each other, and skilled in both motor coordination and cooperation.

WALKING ORDERS

> Locomotion, not cognition, must be the starting point for the study of perceptual activity. Or more strictly, cognition should not be set off from locomotion, along the lines of a division between head and heels, since walking is itself a form of circumambulatory knowing . . . Indeed it could be said that walking is a highly intelligent activity. This intelligence, however, is not located exclusively in the head but is distributed throughout the entire field of relations comprised by the presence of the human being in the inhabited world.
>
> (Ingold 2004:331)

That afternoon, as I am preparing to run some errands, I hesitate between driving or walking to the various stores I need to visit. While Baudrillard (1989) suggests that driving is an interesting medium through which one can understand America, the relatively small size of Haifa, the quality of its public transport system, and its pedestrian-friendly design suggests other modes of locomotion. As philosophers, poets, situationists, and social scientists of various stripes reveal from the streets of many cities, there are many other reasons why walking is an especially useful method to orient our understanding of a particular space (see Ingold and Vergunst 2008; Jenks and Neves 2000; Middleton 2010). First, walking involves the entire body and engages most of the senses. As Mags and colleagues (Mags et al. 2007:201) point out: "the city is not simply a static visual object, it is a dynamic blend of the built, the demolished, the evolving, the remembered, the sensorial, responding to and changing according to the observer, or rather witness (to engage a less visually hegemonic descriptor)." Since seeing is just *one* mode of experiencing the city, I opt for walking, as it enables me to "explore the significance of 'sensing the city through multiple sensory modalities'" (Mags and Guy 2007:133).

Second, walking is conducive to spontaneous face-to-face encounters that are especially prized by ethnographers. In addition to those, Pink (2008:193) notes that following other people's routes and "attuning our bodies, rhythms, tastes, and ways of seeing more to theirs" prompt the feeling that we are "similarly emplaced."

Third, walking leads to discovering aspects of the city we would otherwise miss when driving a car or riding an underground subway (see Chapter 4). Discussing the importance of walking as an ethnographic tool, Imai (2008:330) also remarks that "one can come across many scenes that are deeply rooted in the local and spiritual traditions of that city" and better understand "how the past and present merge in that place."

Fourth, this embodied and mobile engagement should both logically enhance our understanding of a place, its inhabitants, and our evolving relations with them. It can also, as Wylie (2005:240) points out, "precipitate a certain sense of self," a mobile and physical self who will necessarily experience space differently than a stationary or speeding one.

In addition to the individual and scholarly benefits one encounters during casual walks, strolls, or *flâneries*, hiking and marching have a long tradition as mechanisms of solidarity-building, personality-formation, and patriotism in Israeli history. As Oz (2000:178) explains,

> Their physical and psychological difficulty gave the marches the character of tests of willpower, stamina, self-control and determination. Physical weakness, fatigue (which one could not admit to), and wounds were not considered sufficient reasons to desist from the march; on the contrary, they were often considered good reasons to go on.

As early as the 1920s, Jewish educators understood that social, political, therapeutic, intellectual, and psychological objectives could be reached simply by encouraging young people to walk together under difficult conditions in the country's deserts, hills, and valleys. Still popular in Israel today, these excursions—which often include *in situ* lessons in geology, botany, and history—accelerate the transformation of the wandering Jew into the marching Sabra.

But walking together accomplishes other political purposes in addition to just identity-transformation and ideological reproduction. As Ben David notes (1997:140), "In the act of hiking both the individual and the group mark out territory, claiming possession by use of the body—that is, by the act of walking." More radical political goals can be reached faster by marching. For example, well-advertised organized marches to and through the Green Line[5] comprised a popular political tool deployed by the messianic-Zionist group Gush Emunim (Block of the Faithful) when it emerged in the mid-1970s. Guided by a map that uncompromisingly assigned divine significance and rightful ownership to a territory they called "Greater Israel" (see Ben David 1997; Sprinzak 1987; Weissbrod 1982, 1996), the first marches followed in the footsteps of founding members who had previously established legally ambiguous "wild settlements" in Judea–Samaria. As unfolding events later revealed, physically crossing the symbolic Green Line accelerated participants' decisions to cross political, moral, and legal ones as well, and to trample over a fragile coexistence with Palestinians. Today, it seems that these marches have led participants to the minefield of terrorism against Palestinians and violent confrontations with the Israeli army.

If some use marching as a political tool to declare ownership of the land, jogging may also help to reconnect with the past, but in a faster and different way.

Waking up early at my uncle's house in the Denyah district, I decide to go for a jog in the surrounding hills. I trot along the last street of the sleepy neighborhood and reach a wild area crisscrossed by narrow slanted paths hidden underneath intermittent patches of tall grass and rocks of various sizes, shapes, and colors. The terrain is difficult, and I stumble on a number of occasions, sending my iPod flying in the grass. After a while, I pick up speed by slanting my body and racing feet to the contours of the twisting paths that climb steeply uphill, not quite sure where they are taking me. By the time I reach the top of the hill, I am in the proverbial "zone" and feel I can jog for ever.

Looking to the left, I suddenly see them. There! Across the *wadi*! The caves of Mount Carmel Man. I stop. My heart is pumping fast. I struggle to catch my breath. I turn off my iPod and wipe away the sweat stinging my eyes. This site seems to require respectful silence and clear vision. A long time ago, I read a book chapter about archeological finds in those caves (see also Garrod 1962), and remember a black-and-white picture depicting the vista Mount Carmel Man must have gazed at from this location—the azure Mediterranean. As I am walking in small circles, trying to bring my heart rate back to normal, I am also trying to explain my mysteriously reaching this site. Since I have never been here before, I contemplate the strange yet compelling idea that some sort of genetic memory is running through my body and "naturally" propelled my feet to its source. I was just hurrying after them, unthinkingly allowing them to transport me to this site that traces a direct and visible path to our prehistoric origins. Or maybe it's the heat? The sun is rapidly climbing in the sky and the temperature is rising. I am wet, sticky, thirsty, and a bit dizzy. Time to head back to the house, the present, and the rational. But a loud chorus of crickets invites me to reconsider. I sit on a large flat rock and gaze at the sea in the distance, imagining the same place at another time.

WORKING BODIES

> Boots and shoes . . . imprison the foot, constricting its freedom of movement and blunting its sense of touch.
>
> (Ingold 2004:319)

> The individual body and the social body are closely interrelated, both being ordered according to the same principles.
>
> (Alex 2008:539)

Israeli friends have invited me to a dinner party and I am wondering about proper attire. In contrast to the sober and serious clothes adults typically wore in Europe, here everybody seems to be wearing comfortable T-shirts, short-sleeved shirts, shorts, jeans, and skirts. While such clothing is adapted to this area's warm climate, Oz (2000:231–232) explains the ideological codes behind the Sabra style:

> the pioneer's dress had a Tolstoyan quality to it. Poor and worn-out, sometimes demonstratively so, clothing implicitly denoted the removal of social masks, the purity of one's values, and spirituality . . . these were the symbols of the proletariat . . . khaki and blue shirts (worn de rigueur outside the pants) were made of rough cloth of a uniform and austere shade and expressed simplicity, modesty, and idealism.

The same pertains to footwear—a seemingly trivial piece of clothing. Instead of the complex and constantly changing European hierarchy of shoes that establish "distinction," Israelis are walking in simple sandals (called "biblical") or—especially in the kibbutz—just barefoot. As Oz (2000:233) notes, however, this style similarly carries ideological assumptions as "bare feet also meant unmediated contact with the land," and "absorbing the spirit of the Land of Israel through the soles of the feet."

While the European sensory orientation we grew up with required the body to be modestly hidden and the libido to be staunchly repressed, Israelis seemed completely at ease with both, proudly displaying the first and frequently commenting on the second. As Biale (1992:284) explains, this disposition toward the body and sexuality embodied ideological principles:

> Zionism promised an erotic revolution for the Jews: the creation of a virile New Hebrew Man as well as rejection of the inequality of women in traditional Judaism in favor of full equality between the sexes in all spheres of life. For the early Zionists, Oriental Palestine promised liberation of the senses from the suffocation of Europe, suffocation at once traditional and bourgeois.

In a famous speech at the Second Zionist Congress of 1898, Max Nordau, a key Zionist philosopher, was quite explicit about the necessity to forge new bodies for the project of nation-building and identity-transformation:

> In the narrow Jewish street our poor limbs soon forgot their carefree movements. In the dimness of sunless houses, our eyes began to blink shyly. The fear of constant persecution turned our powerful voices into frightened whispers . . . Let us take up our oldest traditions. Let us once more become deep chested, sturdy, sharp-eyed men.
>
> (Quoted in Presner 2003:282)

Rather than hiding and repressing the body, the Zionist sensory orientation sculpted it as a vehicle of work, warfare, prowess, and pleasure. As Nederveen

Pieterse (1993:38) remarks, "First, in the iconography of the young state, emerged the body type of David, the wiry Kibbutzim character, embodying the 'youth' of the Israeli state project." Hazan (2001:13–14) also explains that "The body became visible in almost all of the myths of national redemption: the glorification of youth, militarism, fertility, birth, and death (particularly in battle) . . . The cultural space of Zionism was a territory populated by bodies of workers, soldiers, and brave wives and mothers."

Commenting on posture, for example, Jackson (1983:329) suggests that "uprighteness . . . may be said to define a psychophysical relationship with the world." Changing posture and body use changes this relation and hence may "induce new experiences and provokes new ideas" (1983:334), but also a new self, and hence new social and psychological possibilities. In the Zionist sensory orientation, the Diaspora meant more than exile or geographical "dispersion" (that is, the Jewish people are dispersed among the nations). It also translated into an inner dispersion between mind and body. Hence, the "territorialization" (Boyarin 1997:218) of Jewish identity also entailed the "suturing" of this inner fragmentation, and an evolutionary symbiosis that consisted in grafting an emancipated Jewish mind onto an emancipated Jewish body, growing on Israeli soil, in an Israeli social body. The arduous cultivation of the land succinctly synthesized by the slogan "making the desert bloom" was not solely an agricultural project but also a social and psychological one. Through those geographical, physical, social, and psychological "moves," the people of the book would once again become the people of the body.

TOUCHING INTERACTIONS

> [T]ouch differs from the other modalities of perception in one important respect—it is always a mutual experience: "whatever you touch, touches you too" . . . this aspect makes touch a prominent sense for close relationships, such as love and aggression, while at the same its absence makes for social boundaries and exclusion.
>
> (Alex 2008:23)

Attending the dinner organized by my friends, I try to calibrate my habits concerning personal space and appropriate touching as they gently nudge me to remember that Israelis stand much closer to you than Europeans or Americans, and often touch your body when conversing. Touching is key to apprehend the world, to establish identity, and to define social relations. As Jutte (2005) remarks, it has often been positioned at the top of the hierarchy of the senses in various periods and cultures. This positioning should hardly be surprising as touch gives us a constant and unmediated contact with the physical world, others, and ourselves. But beyond the immediate psychological, biological, and neural reasons explaining this privileged position, touching and gesturing convey ideological messages as well. Gabriele (2008:538), for example, discusses the political comrades' "shoulder-to-shoulder" stance during elections: "this close touching conveys a sense of brotherhood, demonstrating unity and equality among party members, by drawing on a tactile gesture that is otherwise restricted to close male friends." Similarly, Zamponi's (1997:112–113) extensive study of "fascist spectacles" in Mussolini's Italy provides more extreme examples of the gestural embodiment of ideology:

> For Wasserman, the perfect Roman salute showed the fascist's decisive spirit, firmness, seriousness, and acknowledgment and acceptance of the regime's hierarchical structure. Therefore, the salute was an unfailing proof of fascist character . . . Within this interpretive frame, shaking hands was naturally considered a disgrace, a real betrayal of fascist principles . . . Even official photographs of visiting dignitaries were touched up so as not to show them shaking hands.

The Zionist sensory order also entails "commonsensical" haptic and gestural performances of daily interaction rituals. The first step in this reorientation invited European immigrants to abandon Diasporic etiquette and manners, which were deemed bourgeois (see Oz 2000). Released from the past, the new Israeli body could now develop the suppleness and flexibility necessary to manipulate space more assertively, to touch others more spontaneously, and to gesture equalitarian relations more confidently. In the Zionist sensory order, closing the socioeconomic gap between classes, gender, and cultural groups could be aided by bridging the physical space between interacting citizens. This equation is not as naive as it may sound, and as Gabriele (2008:539) notes,

> The social body of the community is mediated via individual bodies. The lived experience of touch, the sensual experience of proximity, of skin and warmth, in combination with the meaning inherent to different tactile encounters, helps the individual to construct abstract principles and classify social relations. Through touch these classifications and the emotions encapsulated in the relations they entail are individually felt.

After the dinner is over, two friends drive me to Tel-Aviv's central train station where I will catch the last night train to Haifa. Ronit parks the SUV in front of the station. We lean toward each other and hug for a long time. I open the door, step on the sidewalk, and turn toward the other passengers for a last good-bye. "Stay in touch," Ronit says a little sadly, "it's been too long." I promise I will, but I also know that, in Israel, "staying in touch" is literal and cannot be accomplished via email, Facebook, Second Life, or other virtual "contacts." As they have constantly reminded me since my visit, it requires sustained and embodied commitment.

POSTSCRIPT

Seeking to evoke a particular sense of place and a sense of time, the journey presented here might be unfamiliar to our readers—either culturally or epistemologically. In doing so, the hope has been a modest one: rather than *theorization*, these autoethnographic notes have aimed at *animation*. Animating times and spaces means making them come to life through the folds, fissures, ruptures, and lines of flight of embodied exploration, through the performative power of imagination, through the intimate stickiness of encounter, and through the seductive power of the word and storytelling (Dewsbury 2000; Thrift 2003; Thrift and Dewsbury 2000). Here, more than in any other chapter, our sensory research has tried to engage with the manifesto for a sensuous scholarship that we laid out in Chapter 4. Obviously, we are not the first authors to attempt to apprehend place (beside the studies cited throughout these pages, see Beer 2007; Bhatti, Church, Claremont, and Stenner 2009; Choo 2004; Edensor 2007; Harrison 2000; Heatherington 1999; Helmreich 2007; Panopoulos 2003; Tilley 2006b; Wylie 2002, 2005). Because of the possibilities for sensuous scholarship that embodied geographies offer, many recent studies of time and place have in particular begun to challenge the realist and Euclidean depictions of social environments typical of the past, and have started to push for a more than representational approach (Lorimer 2005, 2007, 2008).

According to Rodaway (1994), sensuous geographies attempt to excite interest in the sensuousness of the world while describing and interpreting the role of all the senses in spatial experience. For Rodaway, the senses are both a relationship to the world and a means by which place is structured and defined. Sensuous geography is therefore the "study of the geographical understanding which arises out of the stimulation of, or apprehension by, the senses" (1994:5). Rodaway's understanding of the duality of the meaning of the word "sense" is especially enlightening, as it presents an important duality or ambiguity.

1 Sense, as in "making sense," refers to order and understanding. This is sense as meaning.
2 Sense, or "the senses," can also refer to the specific sense modes—touch, smell, taste, sight, hearing, and the sense of balance. This is sense as sensation or feeling.

These two aspects are closely related and often implied by each other. The sense(s) is (are) both a reaching out to the world as a source of information and an understanding of that world so gathered. This sensuous experience and understanding are grounded in previous experience and expectation, each dependent on sensual and sensory capacities and educational training and cultural conditioning.

> The ambiguity of the term "sense"—referring to specific sense organs (sensation) and broader mental constructs (meaning)—is also a relationship between the immediate experience and metaphorical extrapola-tion. This metaphorical dimension has been explored by a number of geographers . . . The reason for metaphorical uses of the senses lies, in part, in the multisensual nature of everyday geographical experience and the complex and ambiguous relationship between the individual senses . . . Sense is sensation and meaning and therefore the term "sense"—literal and metaphorical—leads to deeper questions about sense and reality. Therefore a sensuous geography cannot just describe the experience of the senses and their role in the constitution of geographical experience, it must also consider more fundamental questions about the nature of person–environment relationships and what constitutes a geographical reality for a given society (or culture) at a given moment in time and space.
>
> (Rodaway 1994:5–6)

Sensuous geographies of the present day owe a great debt to the legacy of Yi-Fu Tuan (e.g. 2001) and Paul Rodaway (1994), who were among the first to emphasize the profound role in which space and time are lived, constituted, and engaged corporeally. In this way, space and time can never be understood as mere abstractions but rather must be viewed as spatialities and temporalities. Thus, recent research has pointed out how it is a mistake to suggest that people mentally and symbolically "construct" place and time by teasing it out from abstract spatial and temporal entities and attaching meaning to them, as if these entities were immaterial, and as if experience were simply primordial, and meaning awaited genesis by voluntarist action and by the sudden discursive jumpstarting of culture. Our perspective on somatic work, instead, implies that bodies and selves are always "emplaced" in the world (see Ingold 2000), and this incipient being-in-the-world mutually shapes the sensory formation of place *and* subjectivity, of ways of becoming *and* ways of knowing, of ways of understanding *and* ways of acting, of ways of sensing *and* ways of making sense. This approach to sensing as performative activity is well established philosophically. Phenomenologists such as Merleau-Ponty (1962) and more recently Serres (2008) have argued that sensing is governed by a degree of embodied intentionality and intelligence that transcends linguistic reflexivity. Dewey (1934) and more recently Rodaway (1994) and Ingold (2000) have similarly argued for treating the somatic awareness of "nature" as an active, skillful, performative disposition that is mutually generative of selfhood, embodiment, and place.

We can thus understand these autoethnographic travels as a form of somatic work. To travel means to work—it is no accident that the word "travel" derives from the French *travail*—"toil," "labor." To travel is to subject oneself to the elements, to undergo exposure to challenges, to adapt somehow, and to make sense of one's environment by mastering it, controlling it, understanding it, making it familiar, sensible, and intelligible. To travail also means to struggle, to endure, to suffer, to brave, and to strive to cope with climatic elements, which inevitably sometimes results in failure, pain, or discomfort. To travel is also to absorb the fragrances of the world, to shake hands with new and old acquaintances, to taste the earth, to keep in touch, and, in the process, to create place.

7
THE SENSORY ORDER

I (Simon) am sitting in an airplane, flying to Europe, reading a book instead of watching the movie. Every few seconds, a woman sitting a couple of rows behind me chuckles a bit too loudly. I suppose she is amused by the infantile movie, but I notice that none of the other spectators is laughing. Hence, I conclude that she is laughing not only too loudly but without sufficient reason. What are the sonic norms in an airplane? It seems a bit strange that anybody's voice could be considered too noisy, given the roaring of the engines, the clattering of the plastic trays, the squeaking wheels of the food carts, the banging of overhead luggage compartments, the constant ringing of bells summoning crew members, and the amplified voice of the pilot waking you in the middle of God-knows-which-time-zone proudly to enumerate absolutely useless facts. But still.

I try to be patient and ignore the woman's chuckle, but it is not working. The high-pitched sound is relentless. Exasperated, I rise from my unbearably uncomfortable seat, turn around, and look with a displeased face back in the general direction of the chuckle. In an airplane, where all faces point in the same direction, such deviant head movements draw attention. Several passengers look up. Their anonymous eyes meet mine, which I slowly direct toward the woman whose chuckle I find both too noisy and unjustified. The chuckling stops and I resume my reading.

***

Norms and rules of all kinds—from the more widely agreed and explicit to the subtle, unwritten, and at times even obscure behavioral guidelines that regulate mundane times and places—comprise what we call the social order. How we conduct ourselves sensorially does not escape this panoply of rules, norms, regulations, and even laws. Consider the airplane cabin, for example. Social norms stipulate not only the decibel levels our voices should reach but the tonalities our voices should perform. For example, it is OK to play guitar and sing tunes in a subway station or in the passenger lounge of a commuter ferry, but the same behavior would result in a reprimand on an airplane. Or take touch and kinesthesis. No one would flinch at the sight of two lovers walking hand-in-hand up and down the deck of a cruise ship, but the same behavior performed in the aisle of an airplane would evoke laughter, ridicule, and perhaps even censure.

All of these norms speak to much more than sensations, of course, yet the senses are at stake in just about every normative situation. From noise bylaws to tampering with drinking water resources, from inappropriate sexual conduct in public to forbidden access into one-way streets, the ways we move, the ways in which we display our bodies, the smells we emit, and the volume of our activities are under constant surveillance and are subject to regulation. Indeed, because we *sense* each other's presence, we are constantly on guard to ensure that how we sense in fact *makes sense*, given the circumstances. Such are the issues we concern ourselves with in this chapter: issues pertinent to the sensory order.

By *sensory* (or *somatic*) *order* we mean, loosely speaking, those normative aspects of the interaction order that concern the human sensorium. For example, since sight is generally considered the most important sense in Western societies, visual culture has come to play a dominant role in the value systems of those societies. We are not the first to refer to a sensory order (see, e.g., Classen 1990, 1993), but in much of the literature this concept has taken on some different meanings. For example, Classen (1990, 1993) has referred to the sensory "models" to indicate the presence of a hierarchy in the way the senses are thought of in a particular society.

> Every culture has its own sensory model based on the relative importance it gives to the different senses. This sensory model is expressed in the language, beliefs, and customs of a culture. In our own visualist culture, for example, we use expressions like "worldview" and "I see what you mean." In cultures with different sensory orientations one might speak rather of a "world harmony" or say "I smell what you mean." These sensory biases have profound implications for the way in which a culture perceives and interacts with the world. Walter Ong (1982:6) goes so far as to say that "given sufficient knowledge of the sensorium exploited within a specific culture, one could probably define the culture as a whole in virtually all its aspects." While this . . . may be an overstatement, Ong's point that we would gain a truer understanding of other societies if we were to allow that their conceptions of the world may not very well fit into our visualist paradigm is undoubtedly valid.
>
> (Classen 1990:722–723)

But in this chapter we approach the sensory order from a slightly different, and perhaps more sociological, angle and emphasize more openly the stipulation, negotiation, experience, and actualization of the somatic rules that comprise it. After introducing in greater detail what we mean by sensory order, we focus our attention on how the sensory order is stratified in layers of race, gender, and class.

COMMON SENSE AND SENSORY ORDER

A sensory order establishes what makes sense in specific circumstances, and articulates common sense. "Common sense" is an interesting expression. It refers both to a widely shared way of making sense of sensations and to a basic order of sanctioned perceptions, beliefs, and sensations. Imagine walking in busy and noisy downtown city streets and then turning a corner and suddenly running into a group of people, say fifty strong, surrounding a man who is belching a tune through the mouth of a hand puppet. It must be the performance of a street busker, right? Common sense! Who else could sing so loudly and in such an odd tone without being stared down or anxiously and gingerly dodged by passing crowds?

Common sense consists of habitual sensory perceptions. It assumes that a certain sensory condition has seemingly "natural" or "essential" qualities, which make it good or bad, right or wrong, beautiful or ugly, perhaps even civilized or uncivilized, healthy or sick, and high or low in social status. Yet—in spite of our beliefs that these commonsense associations are "natural"—they are inevitably learned (Herz 2006), cultural, and even ideological. Common sense is the key to unlocking the mysteries of the sensory order.

Our understanding of sensory order is inspired by the Goffmanian notion of "interaction order." Goffman's (1983:2) interaction order posits a "body to body starting point" for unpacking the delicate dynamics of the fact "that, for most of us, our daily life is spent in the immediate presence of others." The interaction order is subtle and difficult to isolate meaningfully. It is mediated by the emotional and moral orders: "emotion, mood, cognition, bodily orientation, and muscular effort are intrinsically involved" to such an extent that "we are constantly in a position to facilitate this revealment, or block it, or even misdirect our viewers" (Goffman 1983:3). So too are the dynamics of the sensory order. Somatic rules and their enforcement orchestrate the delicate interactional dance through which we address and redress the emotional and moral order, and typically compromise with the other. They are also fashioned in time and space that include both the immediate local environments (such as an airplane), history and culture, and, as Elias (1978) discusses, the civilization of bodily comportment. Hence, sensory order is regulated through both formal zoning ordinances (for example, policies and laws regarding barking dogs, "fragrance-free" zones, and so on) and informal mechanisms of control (for example, the unambiguous dirty look of an offended citizen). Sensory orders are never permanent, as deviance, resistance, negotiation, and contestation of the somatic order are common, as many studies of deviant subcultures illustrate. Furthermore, sensory orders are never stable. Preferences and allegiance systems shift, as anyone who has changed the way they look over the years would promptly testify.

Performing the Sensory Order

How does sensory order work in practice? Because it is based on common sense, because it mostly falls into the background of our awareness, and because it is so often uncontested, sensory order is for the most part an absent presence in everyday life: it is there, but you would not know it until it is disturbed, until it suddenly comes to life like thunder on a sunny day, annoying laughter screeching through a numbing wall of white noise, a sudden noxious smell in your living room. And it is precisely these disturbances that allow us to understand how sensory order is performed, how it is constituted and brought to life. Disturbances are important acts, sensory acts that reveal the sensory order by violating its rules.

By "sensory acts," we refer to what sensations *do*. Sensory acts are moves endowed with dramatic significance; that is, with the power to originate other moves in a complex ecology of communication. They are related but not synonymous with speech acts. Thanks to the classic work of Austin (1962) and Searle (1968), we know that by uttering words people "do" things. But any sensation, not only the hearing of speech, is performative. Sensory acts therefore include more than speech acts. Speech acts are always symbolic; that is, their meanings are based on conventions that stipulate the abstract meaning of words and other utterances. Sensory acts, on the other hand, may be non-symbolic, involuntary, and produced by non-human actors (think of thunder in a blue sky, or barking dogs).

Not all sensations act. When sensations act, and prompt further action or not, is contingent on the convergence of various factors, such as the material properties of the sensations themselves, the auspices in which they materialize, as well as the stocks of sensory knowledge available to the individuals who experience them, find them meaningful, and respond to them. Thus, sensations act when others bring them into conscious and reflexive awareness (see Csordas 1993), assign them meaning and/or affectivity, and respond by manipulating their environment. This is how sensory acts call forth somatic work; sensations never determine human behavior. Sensations always have performative potential, but such potential is actualized only through somatic work.

Sensory acts have an intriguing material property, something we call *elocution*. Traditionally speaking, elocution refers to the form characteristic of effective speech. A skilled orator is said to have the gift of elocution (Conquergood 2000), for example. But more generally many sensations can have elocutionary power. *An elocutionary sensation mobilizes: it is particularly vivid, striking, evocative, and attention-grabbing.* Take, for example, a symbolic sound—like the bang of a starting pistol to signal the beginning of a 100-meter dash—or a non-symbolic sound—like thunder startling us during sleep. These sensations are hard to ignore. We may choose not to respond, but we have paid attention.

As these examples imply, elocutionary power depends on context. Consider, for example, the sonic environment of a rain forest. As Feld (1982) has shown in his ethnographic writing on the Kaluli people of Papua New Guinea, within a rain forest the constant singing of birds and the falling and streaming of water constitute a seemingly impenetrable wall of indiscernible noises. Yet, despite often being unable to see the birds themselves, the Kaluli can identify their presence simply by focusing on the birds' ability momentarily to "lift up" their singing over the sonic background. The "lifting up" of birds' sounds—their elocution—and their cultural significance are the dramatic effects of performance and provide the basis for the Kaluli's experience of its material properties.

While important, material properties are relatively meaningless unless individuals reflexively attend to them; that is, unless they are *minded.* Following the work of Mead (1934), we believe that meaning resides in the response to an act, as much as it does in the material and semiotic property of the act itself. Hence, elocution is certainly an important material dimension of a sensation, but so is perlocution—its affective consequences. When subject to somatic modes of attention (Csordas 1993), elocutionary acts have the unique dramatic potential to "breach" (Turner and Schechner 1988) the somatic order. This is an important property of elocution, which is a way of making a claim for attention, a claim that prompts an emotional response that awaits a manipulation of some sort (Mead 1934; Turner and Schechner 1988). Such is the performative power of elocutionary acts, which explains how disturbances and destabilizations of a sensory order work. This is not everything, however. To understand better how sensory orders work, we need to understand how sensations mean.

How Sensations Mean

Understanding the meaningfulness of sensations is crucial to grasp the working of a sensory order. Our previously mentioned study (see Chapter 5) on everyday smelling and aromas provides us with an ample repertoire of examples of the semiotic significance of sensations. What these sensations show is that "raw" bodily experiences are never quite so raw. What we sense always carries the "genes" of meaningfulness. These are the dynamics that we have termed "somatic escalation" (Waskul and Vannini 2008)—conditions in which the denotations and connotations of sensory experience are blurred into one immediate "commonsense perception," so that sensations immediately and simultaneously both denote and connote an abstract evaluative concept. Consider Ashley's statement: "I think smell immediately communicates to guests if a home is hygienic, or well cared for, and consequently, if the family cares well for itself. Civilized, I suppose. Status. A foul smelling home is totally low class—same with an individual. The consequences of not paying attention to odors in the home could be hygienic/illness and stigma . . . Hygiene and self-respect go together." Ashley "immediately" associates certain odors with hygiene (or lack thereof), and associates hygiene with care for the self and others, class, status, health, and civilization. Ashley is not alone in feeling these sentiments. For example, linking the bad smells of her children with the code of motherly labor of love, Karla (age thirty-two) writes her least favorite smell is "the smell of my children when I tuck them in at night and they should have had a bath—the way their hair smells—it makes me feel as though I have neglected my motherly duties." Indeed, sensory perception is often associated with cultural values (Fine 1995; Zerubavel 1996). As Fine (1995:246) writes, "sensory judgments are grounded in social relationships, face-to-face negotiations, social structures, and organizations." These are value judgments that have seemingly "immediate" and potent somatic significance. We easily perceive odor as *essentially* bad, foul, ill, thus conflating *what* emanates a particular odor with *how* that object smells.

The perception of indexes like these smells has a strong tendency to lead to somatic escalation. Peirce's generic explanation of this phenomenon is particularly enlightening: an index is a "genuine relation" (Peirce 1931:2.92) between an object and its expression; this connection is seemingly "matter of fact" (1931:4.447), "real" (1931:5.75), "direct[ly] physical" (1931:1.372), "unequivocal" (1931:4.531), and working effectively by "blind compulsion" (1931:2.306). Indexes seemingly cannot lie. But in actuality they are simply ideal for naturalizing cultural dynamics. Consider Mary's (age fifty-nine) "commonsense" statement: "I associate smelling good in a personal, bodily sense with being clean, with good personal hygiene. Not smelling good is a big turn-off, not only sexually, but in every other way." Mary's cultural association of body odors with cleanliness, sexual desirability, and overall personal appeal naturalizes a perception by making it seem "common sense." Her statement is a typical example of a somatic escalation: we immediately subject body odor (in this case) to aesthetic and moral evaluations: if the body smells good, then it "naturally" connotes a sense of cleanliness, health and hygiene, sexual appeal, and overall sense of human worth and decency.

Sensory indexes immediately denote not only their source but also their normative moral and aesthetic *value*. In this case, as Barthes (1974:9) points out, "denotation is not the first meaning, but pretends to be so; under this illusion, it is ultimately no more than the last of the connotations (the one which seems both to establish and close the reading), the superior myth by which [the sign] pretends to return to the nature of language, to language as nature." A somatic escalation is, in sum, a process of naturalization: of turning multiple abstract interpretations, deeply entrenched within a culture and highly idiosyncratic, into an illusion that perception is natural and free of interpretive work. This illusion insists that the object and the sense that is made of it are immediate, "common sense," identical, and transparent. As Volosinov (1973:105) has rightly pointed out: "meaning is molded by evaluation . . . meaning is always permeated with value judgment."

The fact that we judge some sensations "offensive" and others "pleasing" clearly implies an order that is bound by somatic rules that are normatively aesthetic and moral. Borrowing from Douglas, we suggest that offensive sensations are those that violate those somatic rules. They are "the by-product of a systematic ordering and classification of matter, in so far as ordering involves rejecting inappropriate elements" (Douglas 1970:48). Somatic escalation always involves the somatic rules we rely on for sense-making. In sum, somatic rules are contextual and diverse; their application is consistent but variable.

Sensory order entails a negotiated structure of *intensity*. For example, we sometimes perceive odor as too pungent or perhaps not fragrant enough. Several informants expressed the tension between their desire to be aromatic and their concerns that the fragrance they wear might be overpowering. Nichole writes: "I like to wear a fragrance that is appealing, yet not overpowering." Kate recollects a near *faux pas*, a close brush with olfactory intensity deviance, involving a friend reminding her of the applicable somatic rule, and her prompt conformity: "I tried some perfume (from a sample my sister-in-law gave me) this evening before going out for dinner with a friend. She said it was too strong, so I washed it off."

Sensory order also includes a negotiated structure of *contexts*: we are more or less sensitive to odor depending on whether we perceive sensations as appropriate to the context. As Michelle (age thirty) suggests, the smell of garlic may be appealing in a Caesar salad but, once consumed, the same aroma evoked a very different response in her friend's car:

> There was a day (way back when) that I went to Earl's for lunch and had a Caesar salad. I was probably 17 or 18 years old. I enjoyed the salad at the time. It wasn't until I sat in an enclosed space (my friend's car) that I noticed that the smell of garlic was radiating from my pores. The garlic smell was even more apparent to me when my friend commented. I felt awful. We both agreed that stopping to get some gum or mints was a very good idea.

We sometimes even deem a normally disagreeable sensation pleasing when its context seems appropriate. As Miller (1997:247) suggests, distasteful odors can be tolerable in the right circumstances: the smell of "strong cheese is much more tolerable than if thought to emanate from feces or rank feet."

Finally, sensory order is also structured by somatic rules regarding assessments of *moral/aesthetic character*. For example, we immediately evaluate many odors as positive or negative, good or bad, and these evaluations are not neutral: what smells good *is* good, what smells bad *is* bad (Herz 2006; Synnott 1993). For example, Jackie (age thirty-six) writes: "It is important to control or manipulate odour on your body when you will be in social situations so that you are not judged based on poor body odour. Strong or bad body odour could be taken as a sign of being unclean or sloppy."

Among the most morally and aesthetically offensive odors are those that originate in the body, that odiously upset the public space, and that assault others' olfaction. As Simmel (1997:658) suggests, "that we can smell the atmosphere of somebody is the most intimate perception of him [or her]," and some atmospheres are apparently *too* intimate, obliging "a selection and a taking of distance." Particularly offensive is the moral and aesthetic character of odors that originate and waft from either end of the digestive system: halitosis, vomit, flatulence, urine, and feces. There is a cultural expectation as to what belongs inside and outside the body, and odors that violate these expectations are considered polluting or contaminating (Weinberg and Williams 2005). Because fecal products are regarded as a "universal disgust substance" (Rozin, Haidt, and McCauley 1993:579), several participants in our study suggest flatulence and the smell of feces especially contaminate moral and aesthetic character: "As part of the long term effects of a broken back and fractured pelvis, my bowel functions can sometimes be impacted . . . literally! This can lead to flatulence. I find it most embarrassing to be at a work meeting or in a small event and to be experiencing this social challenge" (Frank; ellipses in original).

Allowing one's fecal smells to escape and assault the olfaction of others "suggests a momentary loss of control" (Goffman 1963:69; also see Weinberg and Williams 2005). This kind of control—and preventing its loss—clearly implicates the expressive and impressive dimensions of olfactory impression management. "Aesthetic order," as Fine (1995:266) has elegantly and succinctly put it, is "a domain of social order." It is control, and we now turn to the ways in which we exercise that control. To situate control of and deviance from the sensory order, we relate an experience of sound lived by Phillip.

CONTROL AND DEVIANCE: SENSORY ALIGNMENT

I (Phillip) live in a small town on central Vancouver Island, British Columbia. As many would tell you, Ladysmith is not just a quiet place to crash at night but a safe and friendly place where police sirens still have the power to startle and where the squawking of seagulls and Steller's jays are still among the loudest noises to be heard. As the diversity of our fowl denotes, our town is also marked by a unique mix of marine and forest life. On a windy day, you can smell the oyster-ish aroma of the low tide all the way from the edges of the cedar-, fir-, and hemlock-rich forests that surround Ladysmith on its northern and western mountainous sides. Most of our neighborhoods sit on those sides, directly facing Oyster Bay to the east and an amalgam of islands and inlets to the south and the north. Oyster Bay is also where our town meets the ocean water and, slightly above the water, the noisy Trans-Canada Highway.

Many of us head out in the morning on that road to work elsewhere, but many stay back in town, too—keeping a safe distance from what is seemingly the only domain where fracas is not looked down upon. Only one block away from Highway 1, the much quieter First Avenue stores orderly bustle every day with the coffee- and donut-infused excitement of the errand and chore crowd, while more distant and farther up the hill neighborhood streets witness the punctual coming and going of school buses, corner-store-bound teenagers, dogs faithfully walking their retired masters, and lone earphone-encapsulated joggers. During the driest times of summer, a cougar or a black bear will venture out of the woods and treat kittens or garbage cans as novelty prey. Aside from that and the Christmas Light-up Parade's fireworks, most of us need to venture well out of town for our bangs and kicks.

Born and raised in a town not much larger than Ladysmith, I am used to the rituals and practices of small-town culture. But it wasn't until I moved here five years ago that I became sensitized to a distinct and much underanalyzed sonic trait of Canadian (and perhaps North American) culture: the *culture of quiet* that neighborhoods such as mine carefully endorse. On any given day, a brief glance at my acoustic field journal will reveal nothing but an appallingly ho-hum inventory of sonic indications of human, natural (as in fauna and other environmental sources), or mechanic presence, including the raspy roar of lawnmowers, the distant grinding of chainsaws and thumping of hammers, the raucous-yet-subdued walking home of high schoolers, the rolling by of large trucks, the occasional "ribbit, ribbit" of a frog desperate over a lost pond, or the frenetic fluttering of a hummingbird in search of a red treat. This is hardly the stuff of most ethnographers' dreams.

Today, as I walk back home in the dark, I choose to explore Fifth Avenue instead of Sixth. But no surprise awaits me there. Nothing is out of our neighborhood's sonic order. As for the last three months, the rain is my most faithful companion on my lone soundwalk: the tapping of the insistent drizzle on my coat and on the paved road, the steady gurgling flow of puddle water into the catch basins, and the occasional bout of wind that loudly clanks the metallic clasp of the Canadian flag against its pole. Other sounds require deeper listening, and a flight of acoustic imagination on your part. Picture people and their noises inside their private homes and not out on public-yet-so-private Canadian streets. Picture dimly lit living rooms inside small but cozy houses visible from the dark street. Picture inside a family around a table, captivated by the sights and sounds of big city media with their chopper news and pistol tales. Imagine their car, faithfully and quietly waiting its call of duty out front. Picture a wet mutt, fascinated enough by my approaching footsteps to stretch his chain all the way to the fence so as to get a loud whiff of me, yet confident enough to feel no need to bark. Imagine insulated family houses, all sonically disconnected from one another by ample paved driveways, heavy wooden doors—one, right ahead of me, without a functioning doorbell, at least judging by the insistent knocking of a visitor—and by windows free of shutters or loud Venetian blinds. Picture short-lived, infrequent, but regular small driveway gatherings where the sonic imperative of absolute neighborhood silence is briefly suspended: parents discreetly coaching their children into the car as the driver's seat belt's insistent *ping, ping, ping* hails them inside. Solitary pre-teens like my stepson Jacob scoring the soundtrack of his play fight with onomatopoeic explosions. Doorstep-bound nine-to-fivers slamming shut their hatchbacks and car trunks as they proudly manage to carry all their grocery bags in one trip, letting out a soft grunt as their heaving unfolds. Then imagine me, walking amid the cars, shuffling my feet against loose gravel, occasionally catching the curious looks of those inside.

And, of course, listen to the never-ending rock and roll concert of automobile traffic. First, the rhythm section streaming in the distance, humming on the highway—too far for me to determine the pitches and tones of the different instruments' makes and models. Then an irregularly melodic layer closer to me, picking up tempo as I walk closer to the veins of its First Avenue artery and rising as I approach the crescendo of its highway heart. Ironically, in spite of its distant anonymous monotony, the first track comforts me and gives me a sense of connection. Together with the occasional propeller airplane roaring overhead toward the nearby small regional airport, its presence is a constant reminder of regular movement, of life humming on as usual, of people moving—of life stable, peaceful, and orderly, yet full of possibilities. In contrast, the second track feels more menacing and constantly alerts me to keep to the sidewalk as the rolling sound of wheels on pavement grows louder in my ears, constantly posing, yet never materializing, the threat of a daring, scornful horn honk breaching so rudely the peace of my neighborhood.

Sure, winter and silence are blending with each other today, but even if you add a few sonic ingredients for a spring or summer recipe, the overall sonic flavor of my neighborhood will not change much. Give it a try. Blend the puffing and sputting of lawnmowers with sparrows and swallows marking and making a spring afternoon. Mix in the cheerful splashing of children's feet on ocean water down the street on the beach. Remove the howling winds, the teardrops of the rain gods, or the sporadic acoustic numbing of a snowfall meant for somewhere far away on the mainland. For good measure, whisk in a dose of runners panting by, a few prams happily strolled by silent young mothers enjoying a reprieve from their babies' crying or nursery rhymes. On Saturday afternoon, decorate with the repetitive banging of hammers, the grinding of saws, the squeaking of soft-sponges spreading Armor All, and the occasional coughing of an old Chevy in need of a muffler job, and you have *heard* the sonic alignment of my neighborhood and the sound acts that create and maintain it.

***

A somatic order is an aesthetic structure. It points at bodily feeling that individuals and communities desire and enact on the basis of aesthetic criteria, dispositions, intentions, and social norms. It is stable only as long as no infractions—such as breaching elocutionary acts—disrupt it for better or for worse. Elocutionary acts that breach the somatic order commence meaningful social and somatic performances. Our attending and response to such sound acts is a unique social drama unfolding toward a process of redress and reintegration (Turner and Schechner 1988) that we might call *somatic alignment*. In the case of sound, this somatic alignment is directed at harmonizing and rearranging the sensory order individuals and/or acoustic communities prefer.

Any society prescribes a particular sensory order in any given variety of circumstances. Somatic work is the sensuous making of meaning. Making sense is not only about somatically tuning in to the world and interpreting it but rather about making it and remaking it into the shape we wish it to have. Making sense, in other words, is not just about representation but also about manipulative action. A crying child in the middle of the night, for example, is not just an elocutionary sound capturing our interpretive attention and a perlocutionary act striking anxiety in us. It is also an act generating another act: our rising from the bed to attend to the child—either through a sound act like "shhh!" or different responses like feeding—to extinguish an unwanted sound and return the world of the night to the desired sonic order. Somatic work in this case resides in singling out a particular sound amid others because of its elocutionary properties and perlocutionary effect, and then acting on it. By acting on the sensory world, we negotiate and manipulate the somatic order of a particular situation, and bring it into alignment with the ideal.

Alignment can occur as a response to a breach of the somatic order and the ensuing crisis; that is, as an action that Victor Turner (see Turner and Schechner 1988) would qualify as a form of redress. But alignment is not just an answer to a negative state. A breach can be a positively valued act. A loud siren signaling the end of a hard-fought basketball game, for example, can bring much relief to an anxious fan rooting for the team that is ahead. Alignment thus characterizes the state of "(re)integration": a period marked by a harmony that individuals desire.

Stokes and Hewitt (1976:838) explain alignment and aligning as "largely verbal efforts to restore or assure meaningful interaction in the face of problematic situations of one kind or another." But as we intend it, alignment is neither solely about verbal efforts nor necessarily about problematic situations. Alignment can be symbolic, iconic, and indexical, and can take place through nonverbal acts. Through the concept of aligning actions, we can hear how the shifting somatic order is constructed and reconstructed through sensory acts to meet the needs of the moment. With sensory acts, we continuously adjust and readjust the graphic equalizer of the somatic order in response to "actions that depart from cultural expectations or definitions of what is culturally appropriate" (Stokes and Hewitt 1976:838).

Still, the concept of aligning actions allows us to hear the relationship between culture and conduct—or, more precisely in our case, between sensory order and sensory acts—and the alignment between the two. An aligning sensory act is a joint act that enables participants to order their sensescapes and restore sensory order. Sensory acts form part of an ongoing negotiation process whereby we fit and merge separate lines of action. As a form of joint action, sensory action is negotiated: we can interrupt, abandon, transform, misunderstand, or disagree on it. Moreover, sensory action can give birth to new sonic situations that lack a preexisting somatic order. Negotiation is sometimes possible, and sometimes less so. For example, Phillip eventually left his neighborhood because—believe it or not—he found it to be too loud, and moved to a much quieter island. But such a degree of choice is not always possible where social constraints run deep, a topic we discuss in the next section.

SENSORY STIGMA

Thus far, we have presented sensory order as a rather malleable entity. After all, we are not powerless and we do play key roles in shaping the lifeworlds in which we live. However, in many circumstances, we experience the weight of culture as incapacitating and the force of somatic rules as inflexible. In those cases, those individuals and groups who are alleged to offend the sensory order have to live with the *stigma* that their sensory deviance causes, and suffer the consequences of their social position. Social life is rife with examples of these sensory imbalances in social justice, imbalances that very often intersect with class, race, ethnicity, gender, and other types of social position.

Alex's (2008) discussion of the politics of touch in India, for example, shows that the sense of touch is embedded into social relations marked by inclusion and exclusion. Caste, gender, and age matter greatly in Indian society, and, according to Alex, touch plays a key role in acknowledging, reinforcing, and experiencing the structural weight of these social markers:

> In the South Asian context, touch has a specific significance, since it is believed to be capable of transmitting both polluting and purifying qualities. The term "Untouchable" finds its origin in this concept, and even though the word itself is of rather recent origin, the phenomenon of polluting by touch dates back much further. "Untouchability" has often been described as one of the key concepts of Indian social structure. The use of this term for the classification of social groups goes back to Sir Herbert Risley's efforts to categorise and stratify low-caste groups in the 1901 Census of India . . . but it has its correspondence in the Sanskrit term

aprishya shudra, meaning "the not-to-be-touched Shudra." In the process of the administrative categorisation of caste communities, the term "untouchable" was used as first a social and then a political category, but the concept behind "untouchability" can be located in the religious realm, where it rests on the assumption of ritual defilement in combination with status. In the *Dharmashastra*s a number of passages lay out rules of defilement, clearly stating which encounter is polluting and to what extent. In these passages the physical touch between two bodies is explicitly mentioned, but pollution can also be transmitted by indirect touch, e.g. by touching something that has been touched by somebody else, by polluting substances or body parts. Not only was the shadow of a lower caste person supposed to cause pollution, but the view is also seen as a kind of touch, of which the "evil eye" constitutes the most extreme form.

(Alex 2008:526–527)

During the Middle Ages, for instance, it was believed that sorcerers and heretics could be detected by their foul odor (Summers 1956:44). Even Doctor Seuss (1957:n.p.) wrote of the Grinch, "The three words that best describe you are stink, stank, and stunk." In medieval Europe, one of the most widely accepted theories of the cause of the plague was the pathogenic odor of putrefaction (Classen, Howes, and Synnott 1993). And Martin Luther seemingly agreed: contagion "poisoned the air or otherwise infected the poor people by their breath and injected the moral poison into their bodies" (quoted in Norton 1975:20). Clearly, "stinkers" and the foul stench of the unpleasant represent constructions of bad smell as contamination of moral and aesthetic character. In fact, Shakespeare's Sonnet 69 (Booth 1977) vividly likens moral decay to foul odor:

To thy fair flower add the rank smell of weeds
But why thy odour matches not thy show
The soil is this—that thos dost common grow.

Such moral and aesthetic judgments were equally apparent in the data we collected on smell. "I don't want to smell in public! I think it is humiliating to smell bad"—vividly remarks Beth (age thirty-one). Indeed, as several informants reveal in their own words, "particular odors, whether real or alleged, are sometimes used as indicants of the moral purity of particular individuals and groups within the social order, the consequences of which are indeed real" (Largey and Watson 1972:1022). In short, an odorous body is an offensive body (Hyde 2006) and failure to conform to somatic rules and maintain expected olfactory impressions is potentially stigmatizing. Numerous people admitted to judging others on the basis of their odor, and, as Susan confesses, unpleasant odor results in olfactory stigma: "I find myself judging people negatively when they smell bad in some way—be it their breath, or something else. I don't usually notice if their smell is just normal or pleasant, but I definitely notice when it isn't." Susan's sentiments might well explain why some people, such as Amy, are not so concerned about smelling fragrant but are quite concerned about the possibility of smelling awful: "While it's not necessarily important that I smell *good* I am very conscious of not wanting to smell bad" (emphasis in original).

It is significant to note an important gender dynamic in sensory stigmatization. Women, much more commonly than men, report relatively frequent experiences with sensory abjection and often in association with embodied experiences that are wholly feminine. For example, Allison inexplicably despised the smell of her own body after childbirth:

> I hated the smell of myself after having a baby. During the weeks that followed my delivery I was followed by a distinct smell on my skin, hair and clothes that I had never smelled before. I can only explain it by pointing out the hormonal changes that were occurring in me at the time. I asked people around me if they could smell what I smelled but no one could. It only lasted about 3 weeks and then passed but I am curious to see if it occurs again with my second child. There wasn't much I could do about it because I was breastfeeding at the time and did not want to apply any fragrances to my skin that may interfere with my child's ability to feed well and establish physical closeness with me. I felt irritated and frustrated with the smell but hoped that it would pass, which it did.

This aspect of stigmatization compels us to discuss gender and sexualizing dynamics further.

Sensory Sexism and Beauty-ism

While everyday life puts us all at risk of potential sensory abjection, our data suggest the risk—and perhaps its stigmatizing consequences—is greatest among women. Women more vigilantly engage in active somatic surveillance, which is, of course, a somatic social control. None of these gendered dynamics can be fully understood apart from the socio-cultural and, indeed, political structures of both sense-making and the somatic rules that structure them, in spite of evolutionary and pheromone accounts that seem determined to do so (see Stoddart 1990). The context of smell and smelling provides us with many examples of how a marked sensory sexism shapes the past and current sensory order of the Western world.

For instance, there are many literary accounts of men's enjoyment of the smell of women. Edmund Spenser (1989:638–639) provides one of the more flowery (literally) in his Sonnet 63:

> Comming to kiss her lyps (such grace I found)
> Me seemed I smelt a garden of sweet flowres:

that dainty odours from them threw around
for damsels fit to decke their lovers bowres.
Her lyps did smell lyke unto Gillyflowres,
her ruddy cheeks lyke unto Roses red:
her snowy browes lyke budded Bellamoures,
her lovely eyes lyke Pincks but newly spred.
Her goodly bosome lyke a Strawberry bed,
her neck lyke to a bounch of Cullambynes:
her brest lyke lyllyes, ere theyre leaves be shed,
her nipples lyke yong blossom'd Jessemynes.
Such fragrant flowres doe give most odorous smell,
but her sweet odour did them all excell.

But, clearly, there is another and far more foul-smelling side to this discourse. Significantly, "the Spanish word for whore, *puta*, along with the French *putain*, are derived from the Latin for putrid" (Classen, Howes, and Synnott 1993:162). Indeed, Havelock Ellis (1928:64) cites several situations where priests claimed they were able to perceive whether a woman was a virgin by her odor. Although not strictly olfactory, the full force of these sexist and misogynist beliefs could not have been more clearly stated than in an English Act of 1770 (Thompson 1969:151):

> That all women, of whatever age, rank, profession or degree, whether virgins, maids or widows, that shall from and after this act impose upon, seduce and betray into matrimony any of His Majesty's subjects by use of scents, paints, cosmetic washes . . . shall incur the penalty of the law now in force against witchcraft.

The "scent of women," though sometimes poetically articulated and other times forcefully legislated, represents sensory constructions of femininity as both objects of male desire *and* anxiety. *Both* accounts reveal much about power and cultural capital.

While the perceived smell of women (or, for that matter, men) is one thing, the use of fragrance is another. Historically, the changing deodorizing/odorizing rituals of men and women reflect important shifts in both the genderisms of the West and the very status of olfaction itself. Prior to the nineteenth century, perfumes were widely used by both genders. However, beginning with the Enlightenment, both perfume *and* smell were simultaneously devalued and feminized (Classen, Howes, and Synnott 1993). Certainly, there remained fragrances for men and women, but they became sharply gendered. Certain scents—floral scents, in particular—were deemed exclusively feminine, a classification that makes sense when considering that the floral garden was (and remains) a gendered female domain (Classen, Howes, and Synnott 1993). Sharper scents—such as musk, pine, and cedar—

were deemed masculine; again reflective of the gendered symbolism of "the woods" (Classen, Howes, and Synnott 1993). However, men increasingly resorted to olfactory neutrality: "real men" do not wear perfumes, as these are frivolous and "suitable only for 'frivolous creatures'" (Classen, Howes, and Synnott 1993:83). Yet, much more cloaked, the En*light*enment would have an olfactory influence of its own:

> smell had been increasingly devalued as a means of conveying or acquiring essential truths . . . Sight, instead, had become the pre-eminent means and metaphor for discovery and knowledge, the sense *par excellence* of science. Sight, therefore, increasingly became associated with men, who—as explorers, scientists, politicians or industrialists—were perceived as discovering and dominating the world through their keen gaze. Smell, in turn, was now considered the sense of intuition and sentiment, of homemaking and seduction, all of which were associated with women. It was maps, microscopes and money on the one hand, and pot-pourris, pabulum and perfume on the other. Significantly, however, smell was also the sense of "savages" and animals, two categories of beings who, like women, were depreciated and exploited by contemporary Western culture.
>
> (Classen, Howes, and Synnott 1993:84)

Furthermore, constructions and perceptions of smell and gender often intersect with sex and sexuality. Beach (1965:183–184) describes the aphrodisiac ritual of a Southwest Pacific society based upon the perceived similarity of vaginal odor and fish:

> Men use a red ground cherry attached to the leader of a trolling line to attract fish. After having caught a fish in this way the ground cherry is believed to have the power to attract women in the same way as it attracted fish. Their vaginas, like elusive fish, will be attracted to the possessor of the ground cherry.

As any observer of advertisements can clearly note, such "primitive" olfactory rituals continue to shape much contemporary "magic" (Miner 1956). The contemporary aphrodisiac *is* olfactory, and routinely sold on the market as toothpaste, shaving lotion, perfume, breath mints, soap, and hair-care products. Clairol's Herbal Essences line of shampoo provides one of the most vivid examples: use of this shampoo is "a totally organic experience," which is bluntly portrayed as a truly *orgasmic* experience. However, the link between smell, gender, and sex is not only traceable to constructions of the aphrodisiac, but the anaphrodisiac as well. If desired sex smells good, and if smelling good is sexy, then undesirable sex smells bad and foul smell is a turn-off. As Largey and Watson (1972:1030) note, in prisons where sexual behavior is often regarded as problematic sulfur is used by wardens to inhibit inmates' sexual drive—a practice that reveals much about our constructions of the meanings of olfaction and sexuality.

Certainly, smell can be a mechanism the powerless use to resist and challenge inequities, stereotypes, and prejudice. Men, for example, are often portrayed as the greatest olfactory polluters:

> Television advertising in particular "shows" that men, more than women, have bad breath, need powerful underarm deodorants, have smelly feet requiring odour-eating charcoal filter inserts in their shoes, and they have rings around the collar. "Secret" deodorant, for instance, is "strong enough for a man but made for a woman," which implies that men smell stronger, i.e. worse.
>
> (Synnott 1993:201)

Still, men's smells are dispersed over the entire body. According to Synnott (1993), women's smells, in contrast, are semiotically centered on the genitals—a cultural construction that makes possible an entire feminine hygiene industry that is built on the perception that women smell bad. By using long-standing cultural definitions of gendered olfaction, the hucksters of commercial capitalism have invented a "problem" as well as its solution, which is for sale on the market. This is an absurd situation, considering that the streets are not "littered with those overcome by vaginal fumes" (Greer 1987:64), nor indeed by the stench of masculine armpits.

Sensory Class Stratification

Gender is a dominant factor in social stratification, but it is far from being the only one. Class differences exist in terms of many social forces, and differential sensory experiences are not exceptions. Many novelists have noted that the odor of perspiration denotes lower class and/or low status (Largey and Watson 1972). For example, Somerset Maugham (1930:140) wrote, "The matutinal tub divides the classes more effectively than birth, wealth, or education . . . The invention of sanitary conveniences has destroyed the sense of equality in men." And George Orwell (1937:159) wrote, "[The] real secret of class distinction in the West . . . is summed up in four frightful words . . . The lower classes smell."

Social class often intersects with other markers of social position, such as race, ethnicity, and religious affiliation. Researchers such as Oosterbaan (2009) have employed ethnographic means to understand the ways in which these social identities are marked and reinforced, and the ways in which social boundaries among different groups of people are built by way of different sensory preferences, experiences, and practices. He writes:

> For the first few nights in my small apartment in the favela, I could hardly sleep at all. It was very hot and humid but what mostly kept me awake those nights was the loud music and the noises coming from the festivities

in the favela. I had moved to the favela during the week and the first Friday evening I saw and heard the many different celebrations that mark the beginning of the weekend. The different Pentecostal churches of the Assembléia de Deus (Assemblies of God) had their doors open and I could hear their music and songs clearly. The little shop on the only paved road broad enough for cars and trucks had been playing *pagode* music since the afternoon, while owners of the bars in the main street were playing mostly *forró*. That Friday night I could hear the sounds of *funk* music all night long. The funk music was so loud one could hear its intrusive beat down in Copacabana. Tired as I was that Saturday, I was also quite excited: it appeared to me that life in the favela never stopped for one moment and that people celebrated the end of the work week together. I was soon disabused about the togetherness.

The different music and sounds audible in the favela embodied an assertive identity politics and the preference for certain music was often indistinguishable from the music's ability to epitomize the socio-political position of the enthusiasts. *Forró* was commonly thought to belong to the *nordestinos*—immigrants from the north-east of Brazil who had recently migrated, *pagode* to the so-called "authentic" inhabitants. Funk belonged to the youth, while gospel belonged to the *evangélicos* (evangelicals). Most people who frequented the Pentecostal churches were very keen to stay away from the little bar where the *pagode* music was playing, nor would they dance to that or other kinds of music in public. Conversely, the open doors of the Assembléia de Deus did not signify the great love of gospel music of a large proportion of the inhabitants.

(Oosterbaan 2009:81–82)

As all of these examples illustrate, the perfumed haze of the bourgeoisie and the musky reek of the working classes are evocative olfactory constructions of social antagonisms. Working-class males may well associate "smelling pretty" with effeminacy, while white-collar men may well express disgust with those who emit a stinky sweat or "smell like a farmer": a class distinction emerges between "earthy-dirty" work and "artificial-smelling," perfumed, and/or synthetic white-collar or bourgeois labor (Largey and Watson 1972:1021, 1026). These classist constructions of smell must be partly explained by sanitary reform and its politics.

In the late eighteenth and nineteenth centuries sanitary reform movements began to grow in the cities of Europe, resulting in what Classen, Howes, and Synnott (1993:78–84) have labeled an "olfactory revolution." The multiplication of factories and the significant rise of urban populations led to a truly monumental problem of waste and disposal, as well as a putrid proliferation of malodor. The need for reform was all the more pressing due to frequent epidemics of cholera and typhus, and "earnest reformers applied themselves to the task of recording in vivid detail the filth and stench of their cities in the hope that their writings would help bring about change" (Classen, Howes, and Synnott 1993:78). In the end, the toll of epidemics brought about sanitary reform and, as a network of drains and sewers spread, cities slowly became more hospitable to the senses. Consequently, "foul odours were no longer considered an unpleasant but inevitable part of life; they were now an unacceptable affront to public sensibility, if not to public health, which could and should be eradicated" (Classen, Howes, and Synnott 1993:81).

Accompanying this public sensory revolution was a revolution in personal cleanliness. Indeed, prior to the eighteenth century, bathing was considered more a sensual and decadent act than a ritual of cleanliness (Classen, Howes, and Synnott 1993). Elizabeth I of England, for example, reportedly took a bath once a month "whether she needed it or not'" (Wright 2003:75). The public sensory revolution would come to reflect simultaneous changes in personal cleanliness. However, the new virtues of cleanliness were not evenly distributed. As the upper and middle classes began to purify their bodies, homes, and streets of filth and malodor, they grew more conscious of the lower and working classes who did not have equal resources:

> The poor did not (and could not) separate the functions and odours of their households into discrete compartments—bedroom, bathroom, kitchen, dining room—as the moneyed classes did. Odours thus mingled indiscriminately in the crowded homes of the poor, increasing the revulsion felt towards them by the sensitized bourgeoisie, who had come to associate olfactory promiscuity with moral promiscuity.
>
> (Classen, Howes, and Synnott 1993:82)

As one Victorian perfumer wrote: "Among the lower orders, bad smells are little heeded; in fact, 'noses have they, but they smell not'" (Piesse 1891:32). Thus, for various material, historical, social, and cultural reasons, social class had a stratified aroma all its own.

While the imagined corruption of the poor was associated with filth and stench, that of the aristocracy had its olfactory sign in heavy perfumes. The rising middle classes, in contrast, would find their niche in the sage middle ground of olfactory neutrality (Classen, Howes, and Synnott 1993:83). In this way, the attitudes and labels affixed to the odorizing rituals of the social classes became yet another nuanced expression of this distinction: lower classes use "cheap" perfume; the upper classes support their position through the use of expensive perfumes that function as status symbols (Largey and Watson 1972)—a fact that, once again, advertisers often exploit. Clearly, "the distribution of odours does symbolize the class structure of society, whether by body odours or by the quality and expense of fragrances. We do sniff each other out, literally as well as figuratively" (Synnott 1993:195).

Indeed, the people we studied also commonly associated class with olfaction. Odor is literally "classy" in that "smell provides a potent symbolic means for creating and enforcing class . . . boundaries" (Classen, Howes, and Synnott 1993:169):

> The most offensive odour I recall is the odour unwashed people give off. It's not even really body odour—it's more of an all-encompassing, greasy, unclean smell. I associate this with the rough-looking (probably homeless) people I pass on the street. I actually find this odour more offensive than plain body odour. While not pleasant either, body odour is something I associate more with an occasional hygiene problem. This unwashed smell is worse because I associate it with a thoroughly unclean person.
>
> (Amy)

CONCLUDING THOUGHTS: POWER AND THE EMBODIED POLITICS OF SENSORY ORDER

We wish to conclude this chapter by focusing on power/knowledge to offer a final reflection on sensory order. Throughout this chapter we have reflected on how sensory order is constituted and performed, on how it is meaningful, on how it demands various forms of control, on how it leads to punishment (via stigmatization) as well as to prejudice and injustice (via social stratification). What we have not yet considered is how sensations can be exclusive by way of knowledge deprivation. What feels good, in other words, is not up for grabs for everyone and anyone. Sensory order strongly regulates access to certain sensations and to information about them. This is an important way in which sensory order exercises its corporeal power, and examples of these dynamics come to us from our study on the discovery and use of the clitoris.

As said before, this study revealed that few of the women who participated in our research had been given much information on this sexual organ by socialization agents. Withholding anatomical knowledge—either by intent or through silence—begs questions of possession and ownership. At issue are not only the possession of knowledge but, in some cases, ownership of the clitoris itself and the politics of touch. "Most women's experiences of sexuality are very partner-focused" (Plante 2006:143) and the same may be true of what is allegedly "her" clitoris. As Sara confesses, "it wasn't easy for me to admit that I needed to have my clitoris stimulated in order to orgasm, I was afraid that my boyfriend would be offended."

More strikingly, imagine the surprise of Kimberly and Jennifer, neither of whom knew that she had a clitoris until an unexpected moment when a *boyfriend* discovered it for her. As Kimberly explains, "My discovery of my clitoris happened when I was fifteen. I had been dating a guy for a year and he decided to go down on me. All I know is that he flicked his tongue on my clitoris (which I had originally thought pee came out of, when I was little) and it felt really good." A missing or ambivalent discourse of feminine desire

(Tolman 1994) potentially renders the clitoris the property of others—a part of a woman's body that is apart from her body, "existing in the shadow of and in light of men's sexual interests and attractions" (Plante 2006:128). Indeed—at the age of twenty—Jennifer admits, "my sex partners have used clitoral stimulation and it is pleasurable, but I have yet to explore it myself." Although she recognizes her clitoris as a part of her body that brings her pleasure, she allows only *others* access. She clarifies an awareness of her own denial by revealing that she restricts access to her *own* somatic sensations:

> I can honestly say that *I* have never touched *my* clitoris for pleasure. I have used an object for vaginal insertion by myself ONCE. I felt very uncomfortable, and did not get any pleasure from it. I was about sixteen years old. As I recall the experience, I don't think I ever even thought about clitoris stimulation. I think that reflects how little I knew and understood my own genitals. Almost five yrs later and I have never practiced masturbation again . . . I hope that I will enjoy masturbation, when the time comes that I too will have some fun. This sounds odd, but I plan to masturbate, it just hasn't happened yet. I would love to explore my body by myself but a part of me is hesitant. I plan to overcome that in the near future . . . Thinking about it makes me want to explore it through masturbation—but I don't. Instead I hesitate and put off the experience. Then I feel foolish and naive—which I don't like.
>
> (Jennifer; emphasis in original)

Just as symbolic clitoridectomy can transfer the woman's ownership of her clitoris to others, language and discourse can empower, which is precisely what accounts for Jessica's very different narrative:

> I learned about the role of the clitoris from feminist writers. As a teenager I hung around with liberally-minded, sex-positive peers. We talked a lot about everything—and it was a comfortable, non-judgmental environment that caused my mind to stretch. Some friends turned me on to Betty Dodson's books as well as other feminist works (e.g. *Cunt* by Inga Muscio, *Vagina Monologues* by Eve Ensler, *Our Bodies, Ourselves*, etc). I was blown away by these works. They turned yucky sex ed into something feisty, fun, and revolutionary. They were unapologetic about their sexual lives and desires, and they were kinda bad-ass about it. This impressed me greatly (esp. as a rebellious teenager). They gave me a new concept in how to perceive sexuality—something to be proud of. Most importantly they gave me permission to be curious—they made it *cool* to be curious. They impressed upon me the importance of masturbation as an act of education and freedom (it helped you learn about your body and desires and it kept you from ever being dependent on other people). It was through these

> writers and my friends that I came to better understand my clitoris. It was such a *relief.*
>
> (Jessica; emphasis in original)

Empowered by a timely education on the politics of her genitals, Jessica and her friends redefined the clitoris *on their own terms.* In contrast to an occupied clitoris, Jessica professes profound independence ("I am dependent on no one") and appreciation for female genitals ("I had never seen anything so fierce, powerful, and aesthetic before. That moment changed the way I felt about my genitals—I'm still in awe"), and concludes, "Turning kids off to the wonders of the body is emotional genital mutilation." It is on these positive terms that we conclude this chapter: by invoking, through Jessica's positive story of sensorial empowerment, the possibility of overturning the sensory order in all those circumstances where it works against us.

8

MEDIA, CONSUMER, AND MATERIAL CULTURE

If a cartoon is a ridiculous oversimplification of reality, then Nickelodeon's seven-year-old Dora Marquez succeeds in the absurdity of her representation. Simplistically sketched, Dora and the other characters demarcate a sharp, if not jarring, two-dimensional existence against a vivid three-dimensional acrylic backdrop. The narrow, slavish, adherence to a palette of mostly primary colors disturbs me (Dennis) deeply. Inexplicably, Dora's chief physical feature is her gargantuan football-shaped head and equally massive half-circle eyes that are almost entirely filled by her giant brown irises. Dora is chronically chipper and has lots of friends, but few are human: she prefers to spend most of her time with her best friend, an acrobatic monkey named Boots, and a loud-talking, gender-equivocal backpack.

During any given episode of *Dora the Explorer*, Dora repeatedly solicits young viewers to assist in solving various problems she encounters on her adventures. To accomplish this, Dora provides convenient pauses so that viewers can answer her many questions:

"Do you see Swiper the fox?" [Pause. Dora stands motionless, but blinks twice.] "Where?" [Pause. Motionless. Blink, blink.]

As a parent of children aged three and five, my sociological sensibilities are severely aggravated every time one or the other (usually both) offers answers to Dora's incessant questions. My children watch enough television as it is; speaking to televised characters goes too far—*way* too far. To boot, Dora's voice is maddening—she constantly yells. I've been in loud bars where it was necessary to yell to someone immediately next to me (sometimes directly into his or her ear); Dora speaks like that all the time. It must be a product of the fact that Dora is hard of hearing; she constantly asks her viewers to "say it louder!" Hence a typical moment with my children in front of the TV:

Dora: "Do you see Boot's bouncy ball?" [Pause. Motionless. Blink, blink.]

My children [seated on the couch and pointing to the television screen]: "Right there, right there!"

Dora: "Where?" [Pause. Motionless. Blink, blink.]

My children [in louder voices, and racing to the screen to touch the exact spot where Boot's ball is "hidden"]: "Right there, right there!"

Dora [jumping with her arms in the air]: "Say it louder!"

My children [screaming loudly and now pounding the screen]: "RIGHT THERE, RIGHT THERE!"

I find I must leave the room.

***

Whether aggravating or captivating, maddening or tantalizing, and at times plainly boring, media culture, consumer culture, and everyday life rely deeply on stimulation of the senses. Intent on fueling our appetite for consumption, communication media and cultural industries are indeed in the very business of producing a material culture—a panoply of objects, services, and fantasies—that more than ever before in the history of civilization depends on catering to the human quest for sensuous pleasures. Scholars who focus on these dynamics have long examined such popular topics as the seductive power of images, the merchandising of aromas and fragrances, the expansion of culinary pleasure, the commodification of touch, as well as the explosion of products and services that satisfy and extend our acoustic sense—from mp3 players to cell phones—and redefine the meanings of sensing in the contemporary world. But other interesting practices and senses, more neglected by researchers, have also come to be defined by these trends.

Take, for example, the sense of balance (also referred to as equilibrioception or the vestibular sense): the sense that allows for the perception and regulation of direction, acceleration, and postural equilibrium. Some of the most obvious instances of the use of this sense in consumer culture are typically found in the contexts of personal health/well-being and leisure. For example, yoga—a practice imported from the East and deeply repackaged for the needs and wants of Western consumers—centers on the search for an integrated bodily and spiritual balance. Postural equilibrium is also exploited—through spectacular dramatization—in such contexts as acrobatics and the circus (one need only think about the remarkable commercial success of Cirque du Soleil). The sense of acceleration is at the core of contemporary consumerism as well. From powerful motorbikes to fast sports cars, and from thrilling roller coasters to daredevil sports such as skiing and skateboarding, to accelerate is, seemingly, to have fun and to live on the edge (see Gottschalk 1999).

Or take thermoception: the sense that allows us to perceive and regulate heat and cold. Consumerist practices that cater to thermoception are legion. The travel and tourist industry relies on the marketing of balmy climates and sunny beaches, and of warm waters and winter getaways—or perhaps on soft powder snow and cool, breezy summer mountain resorts. The clothing and apparel industry is equally dependent on needs and wants for the regulation of bodily temperature through comfy blankets and comforters, waterproof hiking shoes, and outdoor sports gear. Cooling and heating, however, are perhaps the most quintessential commercial expressions of a thermoception-based culture. Indoor heating is as ancient as fire, but the modern technologies can now regulate home temperature during the coldest and warmest months of the year with scientific precision, and often with little need for human intervention. These conveniences associated with thermoception are profoundly typical of consumer culture; as is the energy waste that they produce.

Next, take proprioception: the sense that allows us to perceive and regulate our body's movements in space. The narrowest understanding of this sense in the context of consumer culture could entail an examination of the business of physiotherapy, but a broader conceptualization of proprioception that includes all that pertains to kinesthesis soon leads one to realize that all sport and exercise—whether directly practiced or witnessed as a spectator—centers upon this sense. Even the seemingly least commercial exercise in proprioception—walking—is subject to the ever-growing expansion of consumerism. Walking requires appropriate shoes, comfortable outfits, paths or park trails, water bottles, and more. In an effort to enhance the pleasure of solo jogging, Nike now produces special shoes that work with an iPod. The latter plays music and provides visual representations of one's distance traveled, speed, and so on.

Walking may also be a source of pain, which leads to nociception: the sense that allows us to experience and manage pain. Examples of consumer practices and scientific–commercial complexes whose purpose is to reduce pain as much and as quickly as possible are so numerous that we do not need to list them here.

In sum, what emerges from this brief overview is that a social scientific study of the senses cannot be complete without an in-depth examination of the somatic work performed in the context of media culture, consumer culture, and material culture. Such will be the object of this chapter.

STIMULATING SENSORY ORIENTATIONS

> For meaning . . . remains rooted in the sensory life of the body—it cannot be completely cut off from the soil of direct, perceptual experience without withering or dying.
>
> (Abram 1997:80)

I (Dennis) begrudgingly shell out the twenty dollars I'm charged for two small cups of popcorn, two small sodas, and one box of candy that is large enough to share. Unfortunately, these absurdly overpriced snacks have become an expected part of the contemporary movie theater experience. The expense is exasperating, but it is a price you are prepared to pay: some movies simply *must* be seen in the theater. Or so I have told myself on numerous occasions. I'm usually proven wrong, and it is not the exclusive fault of the movie industry. The climate-controlled theater is spacious and comfortable. The exceedingly high ceiling initially makes me feel small, but the dim lighting before and during the movie lowers the ceiling to produce a cozy atmosphere. The heavily cushioned, plush, dark maroon seating with handy cup holders are especially nice—but the theater never provides a holder for the snacks, which probably explains the candied scat strewn about the floor. That, too, has become another accepted movie theater inconvenience: sticky, snack-ridden floors (complete with melting ice cubes and puddles of tragically deceased beverages), which come to their fullest sonic life as you step on them, are as much a part of the movie-going experience as the overwhelming aroma of buttered popcorn.

Much to my disappointment, this movie experience begins just like all my other movie theater memories. Shortly into the film, I start to hear it: *crunch, crunch, crunch*. It's rarely very loud or obvious—not at the beginning. *Crunch, crunch, crunch*. I ignore it at first, but my silent efforts fail with paradoxical results. *Crunch, crunch, crunch*. The more I try to ignore it (there it is again: *crunch, crunch, crunch*), the greater becomes my perception of the sound. *Crunch. Crunch. Crunch*. Directly behind me, I hear the not-so-faint sounds of a hand reaching into a copious bucket of popcorn for another godforsaken helping. I think, "God, I hope they didn't get the large bucket," but I already know that my prayers will not be answered. *Crunch, crunch, crunch*. The darkness seems to make the sound even louder. *Crunch, crunch, crunch*, shortly followed by three smacking sounds—the telltale audio trace of the most animalistic method of cleansing one's salty, buttery fingers—then the distinctive rattle of ice cubes in a paper cup and the slurp of soda through a straw. *Crunch, crunch, crunch* again from behind me, but this time to my left. Then, rapidly, a chorus of hideous popcorn crunching that seems to surround me. *Crunch, crunch, crunch*. Again, I try to ignore the racket, but the battle is already lost—the crunching sounds, not the movie, have captured my acute audio attention. *Crunch, crunch, crunch* from a person sitting a few seats to my right. The tempo is building into a popcorn-crunching crescendo—*CRUNCH! CRUNCH! CRUNCH!*—and my perception of the noise is amplified, heavy on the reverb, producing a nearly ceaseless echo effect. *Crunch, crunch, crunch*. A half-hour into the movie, the crunching has irritated me to the point of irrational anger that is partly due to the sounds themselves, but also to my own frustration for letting it bother me so much.

***

We experience the world, others, and self through our senses: "it is through the senses, and through emotions and feelings that are located in the body, that social reality is shaped" (Gabriele 2008:240). Accordingly, "social bonding is not only a matter of taking on social roles . . . It is enacted between and through bodies" (Hsu 2008:248). Sensing is thinking, and the stimulation of our senses keeps the brain and mind constantly at work—sending signals, representing, interpreting, adjusting, preparing for action, and sometimes acting. An appropriate stimulation of the senses is necessary for the brain to work correctly, for the mind to develop, and for the self to emerge and fit his or her acts with those of others in the endless flow of everyday life. As Geurts (2002:243–244) puts it:

> The web of sensory experiences and sensory meanings in which everyday life takes place, in which engagements occur with other persons, other beings, inanimate objects, and landscapes [also soundscapes, smell-scapes, touch-scapes, etc.] . . . forms a critical foundation for conditions of interaction, well-being, and health.

As research in social neurosciences suggests (Beer 2007; Damasio 1994; Franks 2010; Gazzaniga 1985; Goleman 2006; LeDoux 2002), there are often incapacitating psychological and social consequences when our senses are improperly stimulated and when our ability to process sensations correctly is compromised.

But sensing ("sense-making") is also obviously shaped by socio-historical forces and is "profoundly involved with a society's epistemology, the development of its cultural identity, and its forms of being-in-the-world" (Geurts 2002:235–236). Different cultures thus promote different "sensory orientations"—a term that Geurts (2002:235–236) defines as:

> characteristic ways in which one is led to focus on and attend to others . . . We see each other, hear each other, smell or do not smell each other, touch or do not touch each other—as the case may be from one cultural context to the next. So how one becomes socialized toward the meanings of sights, sounds, smells, tastes, and so forth, represents a critical aspect of how one acquires a mode of being-in-the-world, or an individual system of experiencing and organizing the world.

Accordingly, sensory orientations "represent a critical dimension of how 'culture and psyche make each other up' . . . and play a critical role in a person's sensibilities around intersubjective dynamics and the boundaries between self and other" (Geurts 2002:235–236).

How social orders shape sensory orientations has been a topic of reflection for many social scientists, and their writings provide foundational insights about the sensory consequences of the various social transformations that have characterized modernity: urbanization (e.g. Simmel), rationalization (e.g. Weber), the capitalist mode of production (e.g. Marx), sexual repression (e.g. Freud), punishment (e.g. Foucault), a new relation to the natural environment (e.g. Morin and Kern 1993; Shepard 1992). While the sensory consequences of many of these macro-social transformations were largely unintended, scholars such as Biale (1992), Elias (1978), Frykman (1994), and Zamponi (1997), for example, document that a sensory orientation can also be purposefully mobilized and reconfigured by a variety of institutions seeking to bolster different political projects, economic interests, and hegemonic struggles.

Some of the ways in which more contemporary sensory studies scholars have addressed these topics include research on the marketing of automobile technologies (Sheller 2004), the utilization of portable music players by urban dwellers (Bull 2000, 2008), the stimulation of the senses in film (Marks 1999), the socialization of music (Ferzacca 2006) and food appreciation (Ochs, Pontecorvo, and Fasulo 1996), the aestheticization of nature in urban zoos (Elliot 2006), the discursive reframing of touch in the context of video-gaming (Parisi 2008), the colonialist fetishization of museum objects (Edwards, Gosden, and Phillips 2006), the rethinking of architectural design for multisensual comfort (Malnar and Vodvarka 2004), and much more. Indeed, it would not be an exaggeration to say that sensory research on media culture, consumer culture, and material culture combined probably accounts for three times the amount of research on all the other topics of our attention in this book.

A particularly vivid example of this literature comes from the work of Michael Bull. In *Sounding out the City*, Bull (2000) examines the practices of urban dwellers who utilize portable music-playing devices in public spaces and reflects in depth on the socio-cultural significance of a consumption behavior that has become as popular as eating food and wearing clothes over the last few years. Cities in the Western world seem utterly permeated with people of all ages who isolate themselves from their sonic surroundings by way of earphones. Whether attached to an old-fashioned (by now) Walkman or CD player, or an mp3 player or a music-playing smart phone, earphones plug the user into a private soundscape that effectively eliminates ambient sound from the immediate corporeal experience of the city. But such sensory orientation is not aimed at outright isolation: music-playing devices open up newer, qualitatively different apprehensions (such as visual) of the spaces navigated by the users of these technologies.

Because we do not have the space to review all of these studies, and because we believe that much useful information about media culture, consumer culture, and material culture can be conveyed through our own research, we dedicate our attention to a brief analysis of two distinct sources informing the contemporary sensory orientation: hyperconsumption and virtualization. Guided by insights originating from the new field of social neuroscience, we further develop the effects of virtualization on our sensory orientation and hence the embodied sense of self.

HYPERMODERNISM

> Any awareness of what shapes us and gives us life, any perception of what we are, any understanding of the world—all of our representations—are now to a great extent contingent upon machines. Within our current perception of the universe, there no longer exists a natural order without machines. That is the technological reality.
>
> (Dyens 2001:11)

> The significance of media as "extensions of man" does not lie in the media's ability to extend the sense organs into the external world but rather in the reconfiguration of the sensorium brought about by this technological conditioning of bodily habits. It is the reforming of the perceptual act accomplished by technological extension that is significant, not the extension itself.
>
> (Parisi 2008:309)

Our discussion of the present moment is informed by a number of contemporary French social scientists, who call it "hypermodern." Most prominent among these are Nicole Aubert (2005), Francois Ascher (2005a, 2005b), Robert Castell (2005), Jean Cournut (2005), Vincent de Gaulejac (2005), and Gilles Lipovetsky (1983, 2005, 2006). While the meanings of the "hyper" prefix are varied, these authors still seem to agree about some of its key aspects. Thus, Aubert distinguishes *hyper*modernity from *post*modernity by emphasizing the experience of intensity, instantaneity, urgency, instant gratification, and excess. As she explains (Aubert 2005:14–15):

> By replacing it [postmodernity] with the term hypermodernity, we emphasize the fact that the society in which contemporary individuals live has changed. We place the accent not on rupture with the foundations of modernity, but on the exacerbation and radicalization of the modern . . . The essential mode of hypermodernity is excess, the overabundance of events in the contemporary world. It is this overabundance of events rather than the collapse of the idea of progress that makes it so difficult to understand the present.

As Cournut (2005:64; emphasis added) also notes, the hypermodern can be characterized by "collusion between the temptation toward excess and the means to achieve it. We must acknowledge that if the temptation is this intense, it is surely because our era has provided ample means to achieve it and *actively promotes it*."

Scholars have documented this excess in areas as varied as professional pressures, individualism, innovations, information, risks, competition, communication, and consumption. Since this chapter is mainly concerned with sensing and media, consumer, and material culture, we will focus here on hyperconsumption and virtualization. Paradoxically, while hyperconsumption refers to a desire for commodities and services that deliver pleasurable sensory *stimulations*, virtualization refers mainly to sensory *simulations*. Of course, this distinction is much fuzzier than it seems because: (a) virtualization requires the purchasing of an expensive material apparatus that enables us to go online; and (b) the virtual "network," which was originally designed for information gathering and sharing, has become a central node of hyperconsumption. On the other hand, as we outline below, both reconfigure our sensory orientations in problematic, but different, ways. Hyperconsumption promotes *sensory saturation, intensification, and segmentation*; virtualization promotes *sensory atrophy and disconnection.*

HYPERCONSUMPTION: SENSORY SATURATION, INTENSIFICATION, AND SEGMENTATION

If the key characteristic of the hypermodern moment is the regime of excess, nowhere is this excess more blatant than in its mode of consumption—or what Lipovetsky (1983, 1987, 2005, 2006) calls "hyperconsumption." Characterized by a seemingly endless output of new commodities and services, and a media apparatus whose mantra is "constant and instant consumption," the first facet of hyperconsumption is a saturation of everyday life and consciousness by commercial messages. As Leiss, Klein, Jhally, and Botterill (2005:3) document:

> Global advertising in 2003 was a $471 billion business, more than half of which, $249.2 billion, were US advertising expenditures . . . Although the numbers fluctuate, agencies employ roughly 165,000 employees in the United States and 20,000 in London . . . Promotional communication permeates and blends with our cultural environment, punctuating our television watching, saturating our magazines and newspapers, and popping up in our Internet surfing, movies, and video games. In short, advertising has become an accepted part of everyday life.

In addition, Lipovetsky (2006) suggests that hyperconsumption fans different motivations than in previous phases in the history of modern consumption. It is hyperindividualistic, experiential and emotional, as today's consumers purchase commodities not to feel unique in relation to others but to satisfy fantasies of a grandiose self. In the hypermodern moment, "consumption for oneself has replaced consumption for the other" (Lipovetsky 2006:39). Many of the commodities produced in the present moment (such as iPods, personal computers, iPads, video games, laptops, cell phones, high-tech car appliances, etc.) are designed for private rather than shared use, and enable owners to customize them with increasing precision in order to meet their constantly changing, idiosyncratic specifications and express their "personality."

As television, radio, the internet, educational, commercial, and other enterprises increasingly merge and operate on a 24/7 schedule, hyper-consumption becomes "turboconsumption" and the impatient pampered consumer expects to have "what I want, when I want it, and where I want it" (Lipovetsky 2006:102; also see Gottschalk 1999, 2006, 2009). Bauman (2001, 2004, 2007) has also traced this transformation of consumers' motivation from need, to desire, to wish. As he notes (Bauman 2001:14):

> Desire has outlived its usefulness: having brought consumer addiction to its present state, it can no more keep pace. A more powerful, and above all more versatile stimulant is needed to keep the acceleration of consumer demand on a level with the rising volume of consumer offer. "Wish" is the much-needed replacement: it completes the liberation of the pleasure principle, purging the last residues of reality-principle impediments.

With the new immediacy of consumption enabled by the global virtual shopping mall, the "wish" stage might soon be replaced by the "impulse" stage. Arguably, this orientation is already visible in the recent ascent of texting as a main form of telecommunication—an ascent that is calculated in trillions of messages exchanged last year. For Aubert (2005), de Gaulejac (2005), Enriquez (2005), Gauchet (2005), and other hypermodern theorists, there are obvious "elective affinities" between the hyperconsumerist logic and the megalomaniac tendencies that characterize the hypermodern subject.

A second facet of the hyperconsumerist logic concerns the celebrated intensification of sensory experiences, and, as Lipovetsky notes (2006: 210–211), the very designs and textures of contemporary commodities concretize this aspect:

> Cars, phones, subway cars, computers, cameras, electric razors: their design evokes roundness, organic and sensuous shapes . . . Commodities must do more than just function efficiently, they must awaken sensual pleasures, offer a high-quality sonic or olfactory experience, or provide a more pleasurable tactile one . . . The logic is to suggest function while increasing the commodity's alleged qualities or the sensory experience.

The celebration of enhanced sensory pleasures that are embedded in the shapes, textures, and designs of new commodities is reiterated in the commercial messages encouraging us to purchase them. Thus, an iPod does not just deliver high-fidelity music to my ears; it makes me dance. A cologne does not just smell of sandalwood; it unleashes wild eroticism. A car is not just comfortable and fuel-efficient; it makes hills shake and flowers bloom. A cup of coffee does not just taste reasonably good; it transports me to an outdoor café in the middle of a Tuscan piazza. A deodorant does not just release a chemical aroma that (we are told) smells of "ocean breeze"; it transforms a suburban den into a tropical beach. Under such conditions, raw sensations replace sense-making (hence, thinking), the sensational displaces the sensical (Barus-Michel 2005:242), and hypermodern individuals confront a "loss of the senses" and "senselessness" (Aubert 2005:28).[1] In addition, sense-making is complexly intertwined with memory, and these commodities that promise to enhance sensory experiences can also profoundly transform memory. As Serematakis (1994:8) points out: "Thus each commodity form is introduced through the creation of its own self-generating experience and memory. The latter are themselves promised as substitutions, replacements and improvements of prior sensory experience."

A third facet of the hyperconsumerist logic is the segmentation of the senses, a trend already initiated in the modern era. As Serematakis (1994:9–10) notes, "the senses, in modernity, are detached from each other, re-functioned and externalized as utilitarian instruments, and as media and objects of commodification . . . The result is the privatized sense organ." Intensifying this trend, hyperconsumerism hacks the human body into a multitude of isolated body parts, biological functions, and senses—each of which should be "hooked up" to commodities and services that can transform every fiber of our being, every niche of our psyche, every inch of our body. L'Oreal for hair and Rogaine for bald spots; Maybeline for lips and Cover Girl for skin; Revlon for eyelashes and Renu for eyes; Afrin for nose and Riccola for throat; Crest for teeth and Listerine for breath; Starbucks for the palate and Pizza Hut for the stomach; Pepto Bismol for digestion and Axe for perspiration; Prozac for depression and SlimFast for nutrition; Vagisil for infections and Viagra for erections.

In sum, the sensory orientation promoted by hyperconsumerism includes an increasing saturation of commercial messages, commodities, and services that celebrate sensory pleasures, promise enhanced sensations, and tear the sensorium asunder into countless receptors of individualistic and pleasurable experiences. In so doing, this orientation might promote, paradoxically, a sense of disconnection from one's own body and sensorium. As we discuss below, virtualization invites further sensory transformations that reorient our engagement with the external environment as well.

VIRTUALIZATION: SENSORY ATROPHY AND DISCONNECTION

> The screen that provides us with information about the world's realities is also a screen against the shock of seeing and knowing about those realities . . . A certain reality is perceived but its significance is de-realized . . . The weightlessness of the image induces a sense of detachment and remoteness from what is seen.
>
> (Robbins 1994:460)

> A culture's sensory order is one of the first and most basic elements of making ourselves human.
>
> (Geurts 2002:5)

We experience the materiality of the world and self by attending to the sensations we encounter as we interact with others and with material objects in everyday life. While we typically have little trouble understanding that people manipulate and shape everyday objects, the idea that everyday objects also shape us is usually less immediately obvious. Discussing these reciprocal effects between people and objects, Owens (2007:567) reminds us that: "human behavior not only involves interpreting and manipulating objects but is in turn shaped by them. Generally this process is understood as arising from aspects of the object at hand, such as utility or perceived potential, which prompt certain responses from us."

The second aspect of the hypermodern moment that reconfigures our sensory orientation is virtualization, a term we use to refer to those online experiences enabled by a panoply of devices typically organized under the umbrella term computer-mediated communication (CMC). This panoply includes email, cell phones, PDAs, video conferencing technology, social virtual worlds (such as Second Life), and other devices, computer programs, and platforms we routinely utilize to interact with physically absent others and objects.

Trying to summarize the topic of CMC is a Sisyphean task. The academic literature about it is growing exponentially, emerges from a wide variety of disciplines, and is fragmenting into a multiplicity of specializations around specific technologies, topics, users, cultures, and settings. It is also rapidly changing as the technologies and their capabilities are themselves quickly evolving and merging. For example, the newest cell phones enable audio-visual communication and most can now also perform such functions as emailing, web surfing, photography, voice-recording, videoing, and information-processing that once necessitated a computer or an array of separate devices. Similarly, the personal computer—once a device used mainly for information-processing and -sharing—can also be used for audio-visual communication and a constantly growing variety of applications (or "apps"). Together, these technologies and the activities they make possible extend the senses of hearing, sight, and voice, as well as mental functions. They both epitomize and shape our contemporary moment, culture, and social-psychological orientations, especially since we use them first and foremost to interact with others. While we have written elsewhere about the superlative logic of hypermodern culture (see Gottschalk 2009), we must still acknowledge the disorienting scope, speed, depth, and pervasiveness of the CMC revolution. This revolution is being theorized and researched extensively, but by the time we reach some modicum of understanding, it has already transformed itself and us. As Abram remarks (1997:115):

> we are simply unable to discern with any clarity the manner in which our own perceptions and thoughts are being shifted by our sensory involvement with electronic technologies, since any thinking that seeks to discern such a shift is itself subject to the very effect that it strives to thematize. Nevertheless, we may be sure that the shapes of our consciousness *are* shifting in tandem with the technologies that engage our senses—much as we can now begin to discern, in retrospect, how the distinctive shape of Western philosophy was born of the meeting between the human senses and the alphabet in ancient Greece.

Here, we are concerned chiefly with the experience of virtualization enabled by the personal computer's apparatus (hardware, software, and connectivity).

Scholars and others have discussed CMC as medium, technology, and environment, and which metaphor we use ultimately depends on our purpose. Here, we will approach CMC as "environment" or "space." Just as a physical space—such as a classroom, a strip joint, an elevator, or a prison cell—shapes its occupants' sensory orientations and psychosocial dispositions, the software, hardware, keyboard, screen, and the other components that constitute the CMC apparatus have similar effects. As Suler (1996) puts it, "when they power up their computers, launch a program, write e-mail, or log onto their online service, users often feel—consciously or subconsciously—that they are entering a 'place' or 'space' that is filled with a wide array of meanings and purposes."

In order to exist in this environment, we need to establish our continuous presence, and we do so mainly by communicating, being communicated about, and being communicated to. The virtual environment is thus composed of an immense number of virtual "sites" where individuals meet, befriend each other, share personal stories, fight, brainstorm, collaborate, and (sometimes) copulate mainly by writing to each other, sharing pictures, movie clips, or audio clips, or interacting as avatars, without ever experiencing each other—or anything else—in the flesh. Interactions typically unfold not between embodied selves but between their visual representations.

By empowering us instantly to contact and read/hear/see/be seen by countless dispersed others, by enabling us to "travel" virtually and instantaneously to myriad environments, the virtual has decidedly excised the mind/self from its physical shell and has given it enormous reach. However, this new power to broadcast one's mind "live" and to access continents of information rapidly necessitates a radical reconfiguration of our taken-for-granted sensory orientation.

Paradoxically, while hyperconsumption aims to enhance sensory pleasures, the virtual environment atrophies and disconnects the sensorium. While the CMC apparatus enables me to interact instantly with countless scattered others, to "visit" an infinity of places, to listen to infinite sounds, and to manipulate objects virtually and remotely, I can participate in it by deploying only three senses: sight, sound, and touch. There is no smell, taste, kinesthesis, proxemics, equilibrioception, or actual physical contact with what I encounter here. One's entire body could be immobile (except for the hands), one could be deaf, mute, could have lost all sense of taste or smell, and the experience would be pretty much the same.

There is no doubt that a great deal of pleasure can be derived from "making things happen" on the computer screen. However, while recent technological inventions, such as touch-screens, enhance this pleasure by providing new experiences of visual-digital integration (Parisi 2008), the haptic sensations the CMC apparatus provides are reduced to sliding one's fingers on flat surfaces, pressing plastic keys, rolling plastic trackballs, pulling on plastic triggers, rotating plastic joysticks, and scrolling little plastic wheels. In other words, the tactile sensations that CMC affords are monotonous, restricted, and repetitive. While the *virtual* objects we can manipulate with mouse, keys, and fingers might be represented as endowed with a wide variety of textures, temperatures, resistances, velocities, weights, sizes, and so on, the *physical* sensations they produce are all the same. Many efforts in virtual reality technology are invested in finding ways to eliminate this disconnect and faithfully reproduce the sensations such objects would generate in/on/against the human body. The inability to stimulate smell, taste, and other senses remains an important obstacle in this technology. Overall, virtual reality fares better in simulating sight, sound, balance, and motion (see Kurzweil 1990; Rheingold 1992).

The reduction of tactile sensations to the repetitive digital contact with plastic objects is consequential for the development of cognitive and physical skills. As Franks (2003:624) reminds us:

> Mead . . . gave highest priority to touch as the primary sense organ in his theory of the act. We now know that the sense of touch and the hand takes the largest amount of sensory cortex in the human brain by far. Mead as well as Damasio conceived perception as a readiness to act, and subliminal muscular movements accompanied perception in preparation for the act.

As research in neuropsychology also suggests,

> language and thus thought arise out of and carry the structure of embodied action, specifically that activity involved in tactile, contact, manipulative behavior. The new field of cognitive semantics makes the important claim that much of our knowledge is not static or propositional but is grounded in, and structured by, patterns of our bodily actions and the indifferent requirements of the manipulative [*sic*] of objects.
>
> (Franks 2003:624)

The social and emotional effects of this reduction are also far reaching. Quoting Montagu, Gabriele (2008:523) reminds us that touch is "like a human need, since it confers security and belonging." For Synott (1993:156), "[t]ouch is not only essential for well being, it is essential for being." As Franks (2003:625) suggests, "the shared experience of the way the physical world responds to our manipulative actions on it remains an important source of intersubjectivity." Accordingly, the reconfiguration of haptic sensations in the virtual sensory order must logically result in decreased opportunities for this intersubjectivity.

But virtualization does not solely atrophy our tactile engagement; it disconnects sensations from each other. Here, tactile sensations are uncoupled from visual ones as the same digital movements are instantaneously translated into widely different onscreen visual events. Hence, depending on the software one is using, pressing a key can as easily translate into an event as benign as adding a space in a text, as spectacular as launching an intergalactic nuclear attack in a video game, as momentarily embarrassing as sending an email to the wrong recipient, or as permanently catastrophic as deleting all the files contained in a folder on the hard drive. The fact that similar digital motions can trigger widely different visual events—with their respective degrees of "realness" and attendant social consequences—seems significant as it completely overrides the commonsensical understanding that different types of physical engagement, pressure, motions, and so on typically produce different effects. In light of the importance of touch, the radical disconnect between (digital) action and the visual representation of its consequences might normalize a sense of derealization and undermine our ability to "make sense" in other ways as well.

A similar disconnection obtains in the realm of sound. Since a computer's acoustic settings can be customized to the user's preferences, there is no necessary correspondence between the sounds we hear on the computer's speakers, what we see on the computer's screen, and our digital motions (except the sound of pressing plastic keys). Thus, for example, we can listen to Vivaldi while visiting a site devoted to Hinduism, or while playing a video game set in medieval Japan. Any visual representation can be coupled to any sound or tactile motion.

Similar disconnects characterize kinesthesia. While our eyes enable us to look at an infinite number of representations from a variety of perspectives, the body remains essentially immobile. By simply clicking on a key, we can move effortlessly from the satellite representation of a neighborhood to a street-level view. In social virtual spaces such as Second Life, clicking on a key can simulate flying or diving, running or sitting, kissing or boxing.[2] While, for most of history, sensory experiences assumed an alignment between visual perspective, motions, and body position in space, virtualization has completely uncoupled these connections. Here, the experience of "realness" no longer emerges out of a synthesis of physical sensations but depends on screen resolution and the speed with which the screen translates digital motions into visual events.

If the virtual sensory orientation atrophies most sense organs, it privileges sight. Every day witnesses the impatiently awaited release of increasingly sophisticated devices that deliver mesmerizing visual representations and "special effects." Similarly, the growing production of 3D movies whose main appeal centers on dizzying visual sensations suggests that we have entered a different phase of what Debord (1983) calls the "society of the spectacle." As Enriquez (2005) suggests, there are interesting affinities between this yearning for visual excitation and one key mode of adaptation to the current moment, which he calls the "perverse individual." As he notes, the perverse individual's single-minded driving force is sensory (not just sexual) *jouissance*, and the main sense organ of this *jouissance* is sight. Perfectly attuned to the screens of hyperconsumption and virtualization,

> the perverse individual is only interested in what is *visible*. His most acute sense is the *gaze* . . . He neither perceives nor desires to perceive what is invisible, opaque, difficult to define, ambivalent or ambiguous . . . In these conditions, the world is something that must be constantly visible and available to him, it does not have to be understood . . . Worse yet, part of reality has been reduced to a generic spectacle that no longer triggers any emotion.
>
> (Enriquez 2005:48–49; emphasis in original)

In addition, the highly solipsistic and customizable visual quality of virtual experiences reduces the possibility of shared sensibilities that are so essential for the conduct of social life, and—as Geurts (2002:239–241) suggests—good mental health:

> a state of well-being is dependent on a person's sensations and perceptions of "things" being congruent with the perceptions of those around him, or that a person's interpretations of various sensibilia be consonant with the mental representations that others hold about those same sources of stimulus. This implies a kind of shared sensibility. And on the other side of the spectrum, insanity involves (among other conditions) a slippage in this area: a lapse or breach in what is deemed sensible, a lack of concordance in the arena of intentional things and intentional states.

Hyperconsumption and virtualization promote a new sensory orientation in different and seemingly contradictory ways. While hyperconsumption celebrates a multiplicity of isolated sensory pleasures, virtualization promotes mainly visual ones. While hyperconsumption promises to intensify the pleasures of each isolated sense, virtualization atrophies the senses, disconnects their operations from each other and from physical sensations. While hyperconsumption segments the body in a wide variety of isolated body organs, senses, and biological functions, virtualization enables the endless permutations of simulated sensations.[3] In such conditions, every person who goes online inhabits his/her own virtual sensorium where sensations are completely disconnected from any referent, and where no two people can share a similar sensory experience of the virtual. In contrast, Simmel (1997:116–117) notes,

> The fact that all people can simultaneously see the sky and the sun is, I believe, an essential element of the union which every religion implies . . . This fact must foster, on the one hand, that transcendence from the narrowness and particularity of the human subject which every religion contains, and, on the other, support or favor the element of a union of the faithful, which every religion likewise contains.

While we believe that virtualization will shape our sensory orientations in ways we cannot presently imagine, we examine below three consequences that seem significant: groundless and nonsensical representations; disoriented chronoception; and sensory amnesia.

Nonsensical and Groundless Orientations

Virtualization offers enormous opportunities for interacting with others, and for discovering and developing knowledge. As Lévy (1997) suggests, when used appropriately, virtual environments constitute primary sites for the development of "intelligent communities" and "collective intelligence." However, one corrective to Lévy's incisive and optimistic thesis is that human intelligence is "part of a biological, technological and cultural whole . . . called *cognitive ecology*" (Dyens 2001:48; emphasis in original). Hence, intelligence must still be grounded in a rich and integrated sensorium—the biological dimension. For Damasio (1994), a neurologist, intelligence can be understood as an organism's ability to produce representations—of the external environment to itself, of itself in its environment, and of itself to itself. As Dyens (2001:25) also explains:

> we acquired mental abilities because the condition of our body has to be continuously monitored and managed by our immune and nervous system. Both systems "read" various bodily conditions and react to those readings . . . But in order to do so, both systems must "sever" themselves from the body, thereby creating, by means of various actions and reactions, a representation of the body as an externalized object.

However, these representations are embedded in ecologically specific niches. There are two reasons for this: first, because "the interactions between bodily conditions and the environment . . . generate representations"; second, because in order to produce representations, "living beings must be able to visualize themselves relative to their environment" (Dyens 2001:26). Hence, ecologically specific physical sensations are the sources of representations, and representations arise in a sensed relation with/in the biological environment. As Mead also suggested, our interpretation of the response of the natural environment is essential for meaning-making (see Weigert 1997). Following this logic, being essentially dislocated, the sensory orientations promoted by virtualization might yield nonsensical and groundless representations. For Damasio (1994:225; emphasis in original):

> Perceiving the environment, then, is not just a matter of having the brain receive direct signals from a given stimulus, let alone receiving direct pictures. The organism actively modified itself so that the interfacing can take place as well as possible . . . Perhaps no less important, the reason why most of the interactions with the environment ever take place is that the organism requires their occurrence in order to maintain homeostatis, the state of functional balance. The organism . . . must *sense* the environment (smell, taste, touch, hear, see), so that appropriate actions can be taken in response to what is sensed.

Because our representations are stimulated mainly by visual simulations, and are dislocated from ecological contexts, we also run the risk of developing representations that are frankly destructive of these contexts. It is true that the internet is a virtual "environment," but it is—to quote Chayko (2008)—a "cognitive entity" or a "sociomental space" that exists only in people's minds and their (mostly written and graphic) representations. It has no concrete physical existence and produces only ephemeral, individualized, disjointed, and simulated visual, acoustic, and tactile sensations. Tragically, the improvements in high-definition simulations of tropical beaches, snowy mountains, and rain forests are occurring at the very moment when these places are disappearing from the earth. Sophisticated programs can artfully simulate the visual and aural pleasures provided by "nature." However, they cannot simulate the often painful, and sometimes irreversible, somatic effects of its destruction—breathing industrial ashes, stepping in a slimy oil puddle, being blinded by toxic fumes, suffering dehydration on the banks of a polluted river, feeling nauseated by chemical smells, surfing through waves littered with waste, itching because of skin irritants, or chewing on tasteless, genetically modified food. Nor can they simulate the necessary somatic work we need to perform in order to avoid these sensations, compensate for their effects, or minimize their symptoms.

This dislocation has additional social and psychological costs. As Gauchet (2005:298) remarks, sensing a firm location in space was generative of a certain wisdom that asked us to compose with our environment and those who surround us. Today, "you can perceive those who surround you as negligible variables. You do not really see them as part of your real world." The routine experience of ignoring the here and now on behalf of a constant "elsewhere" decisively transforms how we sense the physically immediate.

This tendency is perhaps best concretized by the recent proliferation of GPS devices. Thus, rather than relying on our sense of direction and spatial orientation, rather than using our mental faculties, representations, and memory, rather than looking at the sun's position in the sky, street signs, landmarks, or changing landscapes, we now increasingly look at the GPS screen that simulates the very space we are driving through, and obey its commanding voice: "In half a mile, turn left." Here also, we redirect our attention away from our immediate surroundings to the screen that offers directions, instant feedback, and colorful graphics. While GPS devices are certainly useful and probably reduce the number of people getting lost on unfamiliar roads, will this routine reliance on the GPS screen atrophy our ability to sense, orient, and direct ourselves, and our memory? And since "sense" refers to spatial direction but also to sensory and mental faculties, discernment, and meaning, will this increasing loss of sense, orientation, direction, and memory in the geographical space through which we travel translate into similar effects in the social and psychological spaces in which we live?

Disoriented Chronoception

The virtual sensory orientation reconfigures not only our sense of location but our *chronoception*—our experience of time. While chronoception is typically not listed with the more traditional senses, we should consider including it. After all, it permeates, informs, and orients our everyday embodied (inter)actions.

For example, Weigert (1997) suggests that our limited sensory apparatus prevents us from sensing the consequences of our behaviors on the environment, and responding in adaptive ways. We cannot "sense" or register the effects of our actions on the environment because they often unfold imperceptibly, through cumulative effects, tipping points, and over periods of time most of us cannot fathom. Of course, scientists can use simulations to collapse these long periods of time into seconds, and provide visual representations of what they expect to happen in the typically distant future. But these are still spectacular simulations, not experienced sensations. The exact opposite logic organizes the sensory orientation encoded by virtual environments. Here, most visual representations concretize our digital impulses, are immediate, and thus inherently gratify. Point, click, download. As the marketing slogans for CMC devices indicate, the promises of "lifelike" images and of exponentially increasing speed of "response" seem to remain key selling points. Paradoxically, therefore, while the natural environment is real, we cannot easily sense the consequences of our everyday actions. And while the virtual environment is unreal, we can experience them immediately and enjoy the pleasure this sense of immediacy provides. That those actions we can perform in virtual environments transcend physical limitations and physical laws should not be underestimated either, as such experiences prod us to revisit the relation between sensory equipment and subjective experience.

The disoriented chronoception that characterizes the virtual sensory orientation is further destabilized by the dizzying *pace* of everyday life both online and offline. The historian Gauchet (2005:295) remarks, "never has the intensity of temporal experience been greater"; and, as Simon discussed in a previous paper (Gottschalk 1999), this pace can be sensed as both an external and an internal pressure that dramatically affects our subjective experience, interactions, and attention. As research reveals, attending to such sensed pressures has neural, somatic, psychological, and social costs (see Aubert 2005; Cournut 2005).

Sensory Amnesia

> Memory . . . is a culturally mediated practice that is activated by embodied acts and semantically dense objects. This material approach to memory places the senses in time and speaks to memory as both meta-sensory capacity and as a sense-organ in itself.
>
> (Serematakis 1994:90)

The sensory orientation characterizing the virtual also reconfigures memory. For example, the reduction of at least five senses to just three is not just a matter of a simple mathematical subtraction but a qualitative transformation of the sensorium. As Serematakis (1994:28) reminds us:

> the memory of one sense is stored in another: that of tactility in sound, of hearing in taste, of sight in sound . . . The awakening of the senses is awakening the capacity for memory, of tangible memory; to be awake is to remember, one remembers through the senses, via substance.

At the risk of stating the obvious, the memory of eating warm roasted chestnuts purchased from a street vendor in the shopping district of downtown Brussels on a freezing December afternoon is a richly multi-sensorial one. It combines the manipulation of objects, sights, sounds, tastes, smells, proxemics, the feel of the cold breeze piercing through my blue jeans, flickering neon lights, the electric buzz of the crowd, the random stop-and-go of vehicles, the light physical contact of pedestrians one unwillingly brushes against as one attempts the kinesthetic feat of walking through the dense crowd while removing the chestnuts' hard shells. As Serematakis (1994:9) reminds us, memory is a "culturally mediated material practice that is activated by embodied acts and semantically dense objects." In contrast, as we increasingly adapt to the virtual sensory orientation, we might carelessly start to replace sensory memories with virtual ones. As Dyens (2001:36) asks, "what will happen once memories, which endow us with conscience and existence, survive only in databases? How will this transform us? Today our memories almost never originate from our own decoding but are almost exclusively machine-recorded events." Not surprisingly, as cognitive psychologist Clark (2003:4) remarks, the destruction of one's computer can feel like "brain damage."

In addition, the virtual sensory orientation, which, as we have seen above, can cause a sense of de-realization, can also transform memory so that it now includes experiences that have never "really" happened. Since memory (and the very process of memorization) is no longer stimulated by corresponding physical sensations, the virtual sensory orientation severs the relation between the two. Further, since memory is such a key aspect for the continuous project of self-construction and self-assessment (see Waskul, Vannini, and Wilson 2009), this transformation of memory compromises these complex embodied and interactional processes at both micro and macro levels. As Serematakis writes (1994:3):

> Sensory premises, memories and histories are being pulled out from entire regional cultures and the capacity to reproduce social identities may be altered as a result. Such economic processes reveal the extent to which the ability to replicate cultural identity is a material practice embedded in the reciprocities, aesthetics and sensory strata of material objects.

In sum, informed by the uneven and sometimes discordant stimulation of a few sense organs, the virtual sensory orientation compromises our ability to process sensations correctly. Detached from physical sensations, dislocated from ecological contexts, and disoriented in time, it compromises our ability to produce adaptive representations of ourselves to ourselves, of the environment to ourselves, and of ourselves in the environment. Summarizing recent research, Connelly (2010) and Ritchel (2010a, 2010b) among others report that prolonged immersions in virtual environments and constant interruptions by CMC devices negatively affect comprehension, concentration, and memory. But beyond this loss of those (apparently) purely cognitive aptitudes, Serematakis (1994:9) adds that what can be lost is not just the senses but "the memory of the senses"—a technologically induced sensory amnesia and an excision of memory. As she reminds us, memory is also a "sense-organ" that is always intertwined with physical sensations.

CONCLUSION

Throughout this chapter, we have tackled a complex topic with an eye not only to the future of social scientific research on the senses, but also to the future of humanity. The three of us share a deeply treasured friendship that is almost exclusively practiced through electronic communication, so our reflections on electronic media and the contemporary sensory orientation of our technoculture do not come from a hypocritical standpoint—we are fully cognizant of the nuanced promises and threats, the inviting possibilities and noxious consequences, presented by a world in which being "in touch with each other" often means being unable to touch each other. Yet we wish to retain a certain measure of skepticism. As pragmatists, we are neither technological utopians nor dystopians; technologies are merely social organizations whose multiple interconnecting patterns of use can unfold, and do unfold, in myriad ways.

Hence, in this chapter, we have aimed not merely to plant a bug in our readers' ears on our way out of the door. Rather, we have attempted to make an opening, to let some light from future directions transpire into the present moment. We began this book by outlining how the senses are more than physical stimuli recorded by neurons. We stand by that statement. But in returning to the neuroscientific basis of the operation of our senses and sensations we simply want to alert our readers to the idea that sociology, anthropology, and all the other cultural sciences do not stop where the biological sciences begin. The future nature of these disciplines—made mandatory by the evolving sensory dispositions in everyday life—call for simultaneous focus on the *sociality and materiality* of the human world. Sociality is something that sociology and anthropology know how to handle well. But when materiality enters the picture, one can be less confident. As the biological substratum of the human body begins to intersect in deeper and novel ways with the social and cultural domain in which we operate in the context of a rapidly changing technological world, our social sciences must adapt. *More-than-human* sensory studies must then follow the early steps of non-anthropocentric developments in small, but inspiring, fringes of our disciplines.

More-than-human approaches to sensory studies must come to terms with the changing sensorium. First, one key understanding to incorporate into these new perspectives is that neither technology nor biology determines the sociality of sensations. This is why we have not pointed the finger at any one actor in this chapter. To accuse vaguely defined witches and evil-doers such as "technology," "corporations," "the media," or what have you—as mainstream TV newscasts and poor undergraduate essays are wont to do—is blind to reality to the point of being silly. Instead, we have implied that *assemblages* of multiple actors—comprised of complex, and at times contradictory, forces, combinations, connections, relations, and agencies—transform the sensorium, day after day, act after act, experience after experience. This is, in a few words, what we have attempted to express from the beginning with the idea of somatic work. Sensing the world—the idea of somatic work teaches us—is a way of building and reshaping the way the world is assembled. Sensing the world is a way of incorporating it into multiple reflexive dynamics because of which our experience of the world is never static, but always fluid. Somatic work, indeed, is work itself: practice, performance, the very doing and assembling that molds the very materiality of our social relations. Not you, or Simon, or Phillip, or

Dennis, engages in somatic work alone; rather, all of us, at all points in time, are bound together by the socio-material ties—sometimes connecting us, sometimes disconnecting us from one another—that make our senses, and our ways of making sense of our common world, more than just abstract media, and more than just "hardwired" technology over which we have no control.

As critical pragmatists, we view this realization as a good thing. After all, it tells us that we have work to do, and that we are capable of doing it for our own good.

NOTES

6 A SENSE OF PLACE, A SENSE OF TIME

1 First established in Germany in the nineteenth century, Jewish sports clubs play an important cultural and political role in Zionist history (see Kaufman 2005; Presner 2003, 2006).

2 *Za'atar* "is a generic name for a family of related Middle Eastern herbs from the genera *Origanum* (oregano), *Calamintha* (basil thyme), *Thymus vulgaris* (thyme) and *Satureja* (savory). It is also the name for a condiment made from the dried herb(s), mixed together with sesame seeds, and often salt, as well as other spices. Used in Arab cuisine since medieval times, both the herb and spice mixture are popular throughout the Middle East and Levant" (http://en.wikipedia.org/wiki/Za%27atar).

3 The Sabra is often characterized as "tanned" rather than genetically brown-skinned. In other words, s/he is a white person who spends much time in the sun. It is also noteworthy that immigrants of North African origin were endearingly referred to as "Cous-cous"—an Arabic term that refers to the well-known dish of that region, and which has strong sexual connotations.

4 A Hebrew/Arabic word that means "valley," "dry river bed," or "canyon."

5 The term for the 1949 Armistice lines established between Israel and its neighbors (Egypt, Jordan, Lebanon, and Syria) after the 1948 Arab–Israeli War. The Green Line separates Israel not only from these countries but from territories Israel captured in the Six-Day War of 1967, including the West Bank, Gaza Strip, Golan Heights and Sinai Peninsula. Its name is derived from the green ink used to draw the line on the map during peace talks (http://en.wikipedia.org/wiki/Green_Line_%28Israel%29).

8 MEDIA, CONSUMER, AND MATERIAL CULTURE

1 The "perte du sens" can be translated as "loss of senses," "senselessness," and "disorientation."

2 The Wii—featuring games that represent the movements of a player onscreen—is an interesting technological development that bridges this disconnect. On the other hand, these movements do not encounter resistance from physical objects.

3 One possible exception to this disconnect (documented by Waskul 2003) concerns onanistic behaviors one can perform while virtually interacting with others on sites devoted to sexual encounters. Here, there is indeed an integration between what one sees, hears, and experiences, even though one is only touching oneself.

REFERENCES

Abram, D. 1997. *The Spell of the Sensuous*. New York: Vintage.
Abramson, P. and S. Pinkerton. 1995. *With Pleasure: Thoughts on the Nature of Human Sexuality*. New York: Oxford University Press.
Adams, M. 2009. "Hearing the City: Reflections on Soundwalking." *Qualitative Researcher*, 10: 6–9.
Adams, M. and S. Guy. 2007. "Editorial: Senses and the City." *The Senses and Society*, 2: 133–136.
Akou, H.M. 2007. "Building a New World Fashion: Islamic Dress in the Twenty-First Century." *Fashion Theory: The Journal of Dress, Body, and Culture*, 11: 403–421.
Alex, G. 2008. "A Sense of Belonging and Exclusion: 'Touchability' and 'Untouchability' in Tamil Nadu." *Ethnos*, 73: 523–543.
Almagor, U. 1987. "The Cycle and Stagnation of Smells: Pastoralists–Fishermen Relationships in an East African Society." *RES: Anthropology and Aesthetics*, 13: 106–121.
——. 1990. "Odors and Private Language: Observations on the Phenomenology of Scent." *Human Studies*, 13: 253–274.
Amit-Kokhavi, H. 2006. "Haifa—Sea and Mountain, Arab Past and Jewish Present, as Reflected by Four Writers." *Israel Studies*, 11: 142–167.
Ascher, F. 2005a. *Le Mangeur Hypermoderne: Une Figure de l'Individu Eclectique*. Paris: Odile-Jacob.
——. 2005b. *La Société Hypermoderne*. Paris: Broché.
Aubert, N. (ed.). 2005. *L'Individu Hypermoderne*. Paris: Erès.
Austin, J. 1962. *How to Do Things with Words*. Oxford: Oxford University Press.
Azaryahu, M. 2000. "McIsrael? On the 'Americanization of Israel.'" *Israel Studies*, 5: 41–64.

Bagley, C. 2008. "Educational Ethnography as Performance Art: Towards a Sensuous Feeling and Knowing." *Qualitative Research*, 8: 53–72.
Ball, H. 2008. "Quilts." In G. Knowles and A. Cole (eds.), *Handbook of the Arts in Qualitative Research*, 363–368. Thousand Oaks, CA: SAGE.
Banes, S. and A. Lepecki (eds.). 2006. *The Senses in Performance*. New York: Routledge.
Bar-On, D. 2008. *The Others within Us: Constructing Jewish-Israeli Identity*. Cambridge: Cambridge University Press.
Barthes, R. 1974. *S/Z*. London: Cape.
——. 1997. "Toward a Psychosociology of Contemporary Food Consumption." In C. Maurer, M. Counihan, and P. Van Esterik (eds.), *Food and Culture: A Reader*, 20–27. New York: Routledge.
Barus-Michel, J. 2005. "L'Hypermodernité, Dépassement ou Perversion de la Modernité?" In N. Aubert (ed.), *L'Individu Hypermoderne*, 239–248. Paris: Erès.
Basso, E. 1981. "A Musical View of the Universe: Kalapalo Myth and Ritual as Religious Performance." *Journal of American Folklore*, 94: 273–292.
Baudrillard, J. 1989. *America*. London: Verso.
Bauman, Z. 2001. "Consuming Life." *Journal of Consumer Culture*, 1: 9–29.
——. 2004. "The Consumerist Syndrome in Contemporary Society: An Interview with Zygmunt Bauman by Chris C. Rojek." *Journal of Consumer Culture*, 4: 291–312.
——. 2007. "Collateral Casualties of Consumerism." *Journal of Consumer Culture*, 7: 25–56.
Beach, F. 1965. *Sex and Behavior*. New York: Anchor.
Beardsworth, A. and T. Keil. 1997. *Sociology on the Menu: An Invitation to the Study of Food and Society*. New York: Routledge.
Becker, H. 1951. "The Professional Dance Musician and His Audience." *American Journal of Sociology*, 57: 136–144.
——. 1963. *Outsiders*. New York: Free Press.
——. 2000. "What Sociology Should Look Like." *Contemporary Sociology*, 29: 333–336.
Beer, D. 2007. "Tune-out: Music, Soundscapes, and the Urban Mise-en-Scene." *Information, Communication, and Society*, 10: 846–866.
Ben David, O. 1997. "*Tiyul* (Hike) as an Act of Consecration of Space." In E. Ben-Ari and Y. Bilu (eds.), *Grasping Land: Space and Place in Contemporary Israeli Discourse and Experience*, 129–145. Albany: State University of New York Press.
Bennett, P. 1993. "Critical Clitoridectomy: Female Sexual Imagery and Feminist Psychoanalytic Theory." *Signs: Journal of Women in Culture and Society*, 18: 235–259.
Bhatti, M., A. Church, A. Claremont, and P. Stenner. 2009. "'I Love Being in the Garden': Enchanting Encounters in Everyday Life." *Social and Cultural Geography*, 10: 61–76.
Bial, H. (ed.). 2004. *The Performance Studies Reader*. New York: Routledge.
Biale, D. 1992. "Zionism as an Erotic Revolution." In H. Eilberg-Schwartz (ed.), *People of the Body: Jews and Judaism from an Embodied Perspective*, 283–307. Albany: State University of New York Press.

Bichard, J.A., J. Hanson, and C. Greed. 2008. "Please Wash Your Hands." *Senses and Society*, 3: 79–84.

Blumenfeld-Jones, D. 2008. "Dance, Choreography, and Social Science Research." In G. Knowles and A. Cole (eds.), *Handbook of the Arts in Qualitative Research*, 175–184. Thousand Oaks, CA: SAGE.

Blumer, H. 1969. *Symbolic Interactionism: Perspective and Method*. Berkeley: University of California Press.

Booth, S. 1977. *Shakespeare's Sonnets*. New Haven, CT: Yale University Press.

Boyarin, J. 1997. "Return of the Repressed? A Response from New York." In E. Ben-Ari and Y. Bilu (eds.), *Grasping Land: Space and Place in Contemporary Israeli Discourse and Experience*, 217–230. Albany: State University of New York Press.

Brady, I. 2004. "In Defense of the Sensual: Meaning Construction in Ethnography and Poetics." *Qualitative Inquiry*, 10: 622–644.

Bresler, L. 2008. "The Music Lesson." In G. Knowles and A. Cole (eds.), *Handbook of the Arts in Qualitative Research*, 225–238. Thousand Oaks, CA: SAGE.

Brissett, D. and C. Edgley (eds.). 1990. *Life as Theater*. Minneapolis: University of Minnesota Press.

Bull, M. 2000. *Sounding out the City: Personal Stereos and the Management of Everyday Life*. Oxford: Berg.

——. 2008. *Sound Moves: iPod Culture and Urban Experience*. New York: Routledge.

Bull, M. and L. Back. 2003. *The Auditory Culture Reader*. Oxford: Berg.

Bull, M., P. Gilroy, D. Howes, and D. Kahn. 2006. "Introducing Sensory Studies." *Senses and Society*, 1: 5–8.

Cahill, S. 1985. "Meanwhile Backstage: Public Bathrooms and Interaction Order." *Urban Life*, 14: 33–58.

Castell, R. 2005. "La Face Cachée de l'Individu Hypermoderne: L'Individu par Défaut." In N. Aubert (ed.), *L'Individu Hypermoderne*, 119–128. Paris: Erès.

Chau, A.Y. 2008. "The Sensorial Production of the Social." *Ethnos*, 73: 485–504.

Chayko, M. 2008. *Portable Communities: The Social Dynamics of Online and Mobile Communication*. Albany: State University of New York Press.

Choo, S. 2004. "Eating Satay Babi: Sensory Perception of Transnational Movement." *Journal of Intercultural Studies*, 25: 203–213.

Chuengsatiansup, K. 1999. "Sense, Symbol, and Soma: Illness Experience and the Soundscape of Everyday Life." *Culture, Medicine, and Psychiatry*, 23: 273–301.

Clark, A. 2003. *Natural Born Cyborgs: Mind, Technologies, and the Future of Human Intelligence*. New York: Oxford University Press.

Classen, C. 1990. "Sweet Colors, Fragrant Songs: Sensory Models of the Andes and the Amazon." *American Ethnologist*, 17: 722–735.

——. 1992. "The Odor of the Other: Olfactory Symbolism and Cultural Categories." *Ethnos*, 20: 133–166.

——. 1993. *Inca Cosmology and the Human Body*. Salt Lake City: University of Utah Press.

——. 1997. "Engendering Perception: Gender Ideologies and Sensory Hierarchies in Western History." *Body and Society*, 3: 1–19.
——. 1998. *The Colour of Angels: Cosmology, Gender, and the Aesthetic Imagination*. New York: Routledge.
——. 1999. "Other Ways to Wisdom: Learning through the Senses across Cultures." *International Review of Education*, 45(3/4): 269–280.
—— (ed.). 2005. *The Book of Touch*. Oxford: Berg.
Classen, C., D. Howes, and A. Synnott. 1993. *Aroma: The Cultural History of Smell.* New York: Routledge.
Clifford, J. and G. Marcus (eds.). 1986. *Writing Culture: The Poetics and Politics of Ethnography*. Berkeley: University of California Press.
Cohen, E. 2006. "The Broken Cycle: Smell in a Bangkok Lane." In J. Drobnick (ed.), *The Smell Culture Reader*, 118–127. Oxford: Berg.
Cole, A. and M. McIntyre. 2008. "Installation Art-as-Research." In G. Knowles and A. Cole (eds.), *Handbook of the Arts in Qualitative Research*, 287–297. Thousand Oaks, CA: SAGE.
Coleridge, S.T. 1817. *Biographical Sketches of my Literary Life and Opinions*. London: Rest-Fenner.
Connelly, M. 2010. "More Americans Sense a Downside to an Always Plugged-in Existence." *New York Times*, June 6.
Connerton, P. 1989. *How Societies Remember*. Cambridge: Cambridge University Press.
Conquergood, D. 1991. "Rethinking Ethnography: Towards a Critical Cultural Politics." *Communication Monographs*, 58: 179–194.
——. 2000. "Rethinking Elocution: The Trope of the Talking Book and Other Figures of Speech." *Text and Performance Quarterly*, 20: 325–341.
Costall, A. 1995. "Socializing Affordances." *Theory Psychology*, 5: 467–481.
Cournut, J. 2005. "Les Défoncés." In N. Aubert (ed.), *L'Individu Hypermoderne*, 61–71. Paris: Erès.
Crang, M. 2003. "Qualitative Methods: Touchy, Feely, Look, See?" *Progress in Human Geography*, 27: 494–504.
Crossley, N. 2001. *The Social Body*. London: SAGE.
——. 2006. *Reflexive Embodiment in Contemporary Society*. London: Open University Press.
Csordas, T. 1990. "Introduction." In T. Csordas (ed.), *Embodiment and Experience: The Existential Ground of Culture and the Self*, 1–25. Cambridge: Cambridge University Press.
——. 1993. "Somatic Modes of Attention." *Cultural Anthropology*, 18: 135–156.
Damasio, A. 1994. *Descartes' Error: Emotion, Reason, and the Human Brain*. New York: Penguin.
Davis, F. 1979. *Yearning for Yesterday: A Sociology of Nostalgia*. New York: Free Press.
Davis, M. 1983. *Smut: Erotic Reality/Obscene Ideology*. Chicago: University of Chicago Press.
Debord, G. 1983. *The Society of the Spectacle*. Detroit, MI: Black and Red.

de Garis, L. 1999. "Experiments in Pro Wrestling: Toward a Performative and Sensuous Sport Ethnography." *Sociology of Sport Journal*, 16: 65–74.

de Gaulejac, V. 2005. "Le Sujet Manqué: L'Individu Face aux Contradictions de l'Hypermodernité." In N. Aubert (ed.), *L'Individu Hypermoderne*, 129–143. Paris: Erès.

De la Fuente, E. 2007. "On the Promise of a Sociological Aesthetics." *Distinktion*, 15: 91–110.

DeNora, T. 1997. "Music and Erotic Agency—Sonic Resources and Social-Sexual Action." *Body and Society*, 3: 43–65.

——. 2000. *Music in Everyday Life*. Cambridge: Cambridge University Press.

Denzin, N. 1996. *Interpretive Ethnography: Ethnographic Practices for the Twenty-First Century*. Thousand Oaks, CA: SAGE.

Descartes, R. 2010 [1641]. *Meditations on First Philosophy*. New York: CreateSpace.

Desjarlais, R. 2003. *Sensory Biographies: Lives and Deaths among Nepal's Yolmo Buddhists*. Berkeley: University of California Press.

Devall, B. and G. Sessions. 1985. *Deep Ecology: Living as if Nature Mattered*. Salt Lake City, UT: Peregrine Smith Books.

Dewey, J. 1929. *Experience and Nature*. Chicago: Open Court.

——. 1934. *Art as Experience*. New York: Minton.

——. 1967 [1887]. *John Dewey: The Early Works 1882–1898*. Edited by Herbert Schneider. Carbondale: Southern Illinois University Press.

——. 2002 [1922]. *Human Nature and Conduct*. Amherst, NY: Prometheus.

Dewsbury, J.D. 2000. "Performativity and the Event: Enacting a Philosophy of Difference." *Environment and Planning D*, 18: 473–496.

Dobres, M. 2002. "Meaning in the Making: Agency and the Social Embodiment of Technology and Art." In M.B. Schiffer (ed.), *Anthropological Perspectives on Technology*, 47–67. Albuquerque: University of New Mexico Press.

Doctor Seuss. 1957. *How the Grinch Stole Christmas!* New York: Random House.

Douglas, M. 1970. *Purity and Danger*. Harmondsworth: Penguin Books.

Drobnick, J. (ed.). 2006. *The Smell Culture Reader*. New York: Berg.

Dyens, O. 2001. *Metal and Flesh: Technology Takes Over*. Cambridge, MA: MIT Press.

Edensor, T. 2000. "Walking in the British Countryside: Reflexivity, Embodied Practices, and Ways to Escape." *Body and Society*, 9: 164–180.

——. 2003. "M6: Junction 19–16: Defamiliarizing the Mundane Roadscape." *Space and Culture*, 6: 151–168.

——. 2007. "Sensing the Ruin." *Senses and Society*, 2: 217–232.

Edwards, E. and K. Bhaumik 2008. *Visual Sense: A Cultural Reader*. Oxford: Berg.

Edwards, E., C. Gosden, and R. Phillips. 2006. "Introduction." In E. Edwards, C. Gosden, and R. Phillips (eds.), *Sensible Objects: Colonialism, Museums, and Material Culture*, 1–33. Oxford: Berg.

Elias, N. 1978. *The History of Manners*. New York: Pantheon.

Elliot, N.L. 2006. "See it, Sense it, Save it: Economies of Multisensuality in Contemporary Zoos." *Senses and Society*, 1: 203–224.

Ellis, C. 2004. *The Ethnographic I*. Walnut Creek, CA: AltaMira Press.

Ellis, H. 1928. *Studies in the Psychology of Sex*. Volume 7. New York: Random House.
Engen, T. 1991. *Odor Sensation and Memory*. New York: Praeger.
Enriquez, E. 2005. "L'Idéal Type de L'Individu Hypermoderne: L'Individu Pervers?" In N. Aubert (ed.), *L'Individu Hypermoderne*, 38–57. Paris: Erès.
Even-Zohara, I. 1981. "The Emergence of a Native Hebrew Culture in Palestine: 1882–1948." *Journal of Israeli History*, 2: 167–184.
Feld, S. 1982. *Sound and Sentiment: Birds, Weeping, Poetics, and Song in Kaluli Expression*. Philadelphia: University of Pennsylvania Press.
Feld, S. and K. Basso (eds.). 1996. *Senses of Place*. Albuquerque, NM: School of American Research.
Ferzacca, S. 2006. "Learning How to Listen: Kroncong Music in a Javanese Neighborhood." *Senses and Society*, 1: 331–358.
Fine, G.A. 1987. *With the Boys: Little League Baseball and Preadolescent Culture*. Chicago: University of Chicago Press.
——. 1995. "Wittgenstein's Kitchen: Sharing Meaning in Restaurant Work." *Theory and Society*, 24: 245–269.
——. 1996. *Kitchens: The Culture of Restaurant Work*. Berkeley: University of California Press.
——. 2003. *Morel Tales: The Culture of Mushrooming*. Champaign: University of Illinois Press.
Fine, G.A. and T. Hallett. 2003. "Dust: A Study in Sociological Miniaturism." *Sociological Quarterly*, 44: 1–15.
Finnegan, R. 2002. *Communicating: The Multiple Modes of Human Interconnection*. New York: Routledge.
Fischler, C. 1988. "Food, Self and Identity." *Social Science Information*, 27: 275–292.
Frank, A. 1995. *The Wounded Storyteller: Body, Illness, and Ethics*. Chicago: University of Chicago Press.
Franks, D. 2003. "Mutual Interests, Different Lenses: Current Neuroscience and Symbolic Interaction." *Symbolic Interaction*, 26: 613–630.
——. 2010. *Neurosociology: The Nexus between Neuroscience and Social Psychology*. Richmond, VA: Springer.
Frykman, J. 1994. "On the Move: The Struggle for the Body in Sweden in the 1930s." In N. Serematakis (ed.), *The Senses Still: Perception and Memory as Material Culture in Modernity*, 63–85. Boulder, CO: Westview.
Futrell, R., P. Simi, and S. Gottschalk. 2006. "Understanding Music in Movements: The White Power Movement Music Scene." *Sociological Quarterly*, 47: 275–304.
Gabriele, A. 2008. "A Sense of Belonging and Exclusion: 'Touchability' and 'Untouchability' in Tamil Nadu." *Ethnos*, 73: 523–543.
Gagnon, J. and W. Simon. 1973. *Sexual Conduct*. Chicago: Aldine.
Gallegos, D. and A. McHoul. 2006. "'It's not about Good Taste. It's about Tastes Good': Bourdieu, and Campbell's Soup . . . and beyond." *Senses and Society*, 1: 165–181.
Garrod, D. 1962. "The Middle Palaeolithic of the Near East and the Problem of Mount Carmel Man." *Journal of the Royal Anthropological Institute of Great Britain and Ireland*, 92: 232–259.

Gauchet, M. 2005. "Vers une Mutation Anthropologique?" In N. Aubert (ed.), *L'Individu Hypermoderne*, 291–301. Paris: Erès.
Gazzaniga, M.S. 1985. *The Social Brain*. New York: Basic Books.
Geertz, C. 1973. *The Interpretation of Cultures*. New York: Basic Books.
Gell, A. 1998. *Art and Agency*. Oxford: Oxford University Press.
——. 2006. "Magic, Perfume, Dream." In J. Drobnick (ed.), *The Smell Culture Reader*, 400–410. Oxford: Berg.
Geurts, K. 2002. *Culture and the Senses: Bodily Ways of Knowing in an African Community*. Berkeley: University of California Press.
——. 2003. "On Rocks, Walks, and Talks in West Africa: Cultural Categories and an Anthropology of the Senses." *Ethnos*, 30: 178–198.
Gibson, J. 1979. *The Ecological Approach to Perception*. London: Houghton Mifflin.
——. 1983. *The Senses Considered as Perceptual Systems*. Detroit, MI: Greenwood Press.
Gilbert, A. (ed.) 1995. *Compendium of Olfactory Research*. Dubuque, IA: Kendall.
Goffman, E. 1955. "On Face-Work: An Analysis of Ritual Elements in Social Interaction." *Psychiatry: Interpersonal and Biological Processes*, 18: 213–231.
——. 1959. *The Presentation of Self in Everyday Life*. Garden City, NY: Doubleday.
——. 1963. *Stigma: Notes on the Management of Spoiled Identity*. Englewood Cliffs, NJ: Prentice-Hall.
——. 1967. *Interaction Ritual: Essays in Face-to-Face Behavior*. Chicago: Aldine.
——. 1971. *Strategic Interaction*. Philadelphia: University of Pennsylvania Press.
——. 1974. *Frame Analysis*. New York: Harper.
——. 1979. *Gender Advertisements*. New York: Harper Colophon.
——. 1983. "The Interaction Order." *American Sociological Review*, 48: 1–17.
——. 1989. "On Fieldwork." *Journal of Contemporary Ethnography*, 18: 123–132.
Goleman, D. 2006. *Social Intelligence*. New York: Bantam.
Gottschalk, S. 1999. "Speed Culture: Fast Strategies in TV Commercials." *Qualitative Sociology*, 22: 311–329.
——. 2006. "Prozac, Postmodernism and Politics." In L. Rubin (ed.), *Psychotropic Drugs and Popular Culture: Essays on Medicine, Mental Health and the Media*, 61–84. Jefferson, NC: McFarland.
——. 2009. "Hypermodern Consumption and Megalomania: Superlatives in Commercials." *Journal of Consumer Culture*, 9: 307–327.
Greer, G. 1987. *The Mad Woman's Underclothes*. London: Pan/Picador.
Grimes, R. 1995. *Readings in Ritual Studies*. Englewood Cliffs, NJ: Prentice-Hall.
Hall, T., B. Lashua, and A. Coffey. 2008. "Sound and the Everyday in Qualitative Research." *Qualitative Inquiry*, 14: 1019–1040.
Harrison, P. 2000. "Making Sense: Embodiment and the Sensibilities of the Everyday." *Environment and Planning D*, 18: 497–517.
Harvey, S.A. 2006. *Scenting Salvation: Ancient Christianity and the Olfactory Imagination*. Berkeley: University of California Press.
Hazan, H. 2001. *Simulated Dreams: Israeli Youth and Virtual Zionism*. New York: Berghahn Books.
Heatherington, T. 1999. "Street Tactics: Catholic Ritual and the Senses of the Past in Central Sardinia." *Ethnology*, 38: 315–334.

Heidegger, M. 1993. *Basic Writings*. New York: HarperCollins.
Heiman, J.R. 1975. "Responses to Erotica: An Exploration of Physiological and Psychological Correlates of Human Sexual Response." *Dissertation Abstracts International*, 36(5B): 2472.
Helman, A. 2002. "'Even the Dogs in the Street Bark in Hebrew': National Ideology and Everyday Culture in Tel-Aviv." *Jewish Quarterly Review*, 92: 359–382.
Helmreich, S. 2007. "An Anthropologist Underwater: Immersive Soundscapes, Submarine Cyborgs, and Transductive Ethnography." *American Ethnologist*, 34: 621–641.
Hennion, A. 2004. "Pragmatics of Taste." In M. Jacobs and N. Hanrahan (eds.), *The Blackwell Companion to the Sociology of Culture*, 131–144. Oxford: Blackwell.
——. 2007. "Those Things that Hold us Together: Taste and Sociology." *Cultural Sociology*, 1: 97–114.
Henslin, J. and M. Biggs. 1971. "Dramaturgical Desexualization: The Sociology of the Vaginal Examination." In J. Henslin (ed.), *Studies in the Sociology of Sex*, 243–272. New York: Appleton–Century–Crofts.
Herz, R. 2006. "I Know What I Like: Understanding Odor Preferences." In J. Drobnick (ed.), *The Smell Culture Reader*, 75–94. Oxford: Berg.
Hirsch, A. 2006. "Nostalgia: The Odours of Childhood and Society." In J. Drobnick (ed.), *The Smell Culture Reader*, 134–152. Oxford: Berg.
Hochschild, A. 1983. *The Managed Heart: Commercialization of Human Feeling*. Berkeley: University of California Press.
Hockey, J. 2006. "Sensing the Run: The Senses and Distant Running." *Senses and Society*, 1: 183–201.
Hockey, J. and J.A. Collinson, 2007. "Grasping the Phenomenology of Sporting Bodies." *International Review for the Sociology of Sport*, 42: 115–131.
Hoffer, P.C. 2003. *Sensory World in Early America*. Baltimore, MD: Johns Hopkins University Press.
Howes, D. 1987. "Olfaction and Transition: An Essay on the Ritual Uses of Smell." *Canadian Review of Sociology and Anthropology*, 24: 398–416.
—— (ed.). 1991. *The Varieties of Sensory Experience: A Sourcebook in the Anthropology of the Senses*. Toronto: University of Toronto Press.
——. 2003. *Sensual Relations: Engaging the Senses in Culture and Social Theory*. Ann Arbor: University of Michigan Press.
——. 2005. *Empire of the Senses: The Sensual Culture Reader*. Oxford: Berg.
—— (ed.). 2009. *The Sixth Sense Reader*. Oxford: Berg.
Hsu, E. 2008. "The Senses and the Social: An Introduction." *Ethnos*, 73: 433–443.
Huxley, A. 1942. *The Art of Seeing*. London: Chatto.
Hyde, A. 2006. "Offensive Bodies." In J. Drobnick (ed.), *The Smell Culture Reader*, 95–112. Oxford: Berg.
Imai, H. 2008. "Senses on the Move: Multisensory Encounters with Street Vendors in the Japanese Urban Alleyway Roji." *Senses and Society*, 3: 329–338.
Ingold, T. 2000. *Perception of the Environment: Essays in Livelihood, Dwelling, and Skill*. London: Routledge.

——. 2004. "Culture on the Ground: The World Perceived through the Feet." *Journal of Material Culture*, 9: 315–340.
Ingold, T. and J.L. Vergunst (eds.). 2008. *Ways of Walking: Ethnography and Practice on Foot*. Aldershot: Ashgate.
Jackson, A. 1968. "Sound and Ritual." *Man*, 3 (NS): 293–300.
Jackson, M. 1983. "Knowledge of the Body." *Man*, 18: 327–345.
James, W. 1983 [1890]. *Principles of Psychology*. Cambridge, MA: Harvard University Press.
Jenks, C. and T. Neves. 2000. "A Walk on the Wild Side: Urban Ethnography Meets the Flâneur." *Cultural Values*, 4: 1–17.
Jonaitis, A. 2006. "Smoked Fish and Fermented Oil: Taste and Smell among the Kwakwaka'wakw." In E. Edwards, C. Gosden, and R. Phillips (eds.), *Sensible Objects: Colonialism, Museums, and Material Culture*, 141–168. Oxford: Berg.
Jutte, R. 2005. *A History of the Senses: From Antiquity to Cyberspace*. Cambridge: Polity Press.
Kaufman, H. 2005. "Jewish Sports in the Diaspora, Yishuv, and Israel: Between Nationalism and Politics." *Israel Studies*, 10: 147–167.
Kessler, S. and W. McKenna. 1978. *Gender: An Ethnomethodological Approach*. Chicago: University of Chicago Press.
Kirshenblatt-Gimblett, B. 1999. "Food as a Performance Medium." *Performance Research*, 4: 1–30.
Kleiner, S. 2009. "Thinking with the Mind, Syncing with the Body: Ballet as Symbolic and Non-Symbolic Interaction." *Symbolic Interaction*, 32: 236–259.
Knowles, G. and A. Cole (eds.). 2008. *Handbook of the Arts in Qualitative Research*. Thousand Oaks, CA: SAGE.
Korsmeyer, C. (ed.). 2005. *The Taste Culture Reader*. Oxford: Berg.
Kress, G. and T. Van Leeuwen. 1996. *Reading Images: The Grammar of Visual Design*. London: Routledge.
Kurzweil, R. 1990. *The Age of Intelligent Machines*. Cambridge, MA: MIT Press.
Laderman, C. and M. Roseman (eds.). 1996. *The Performance of Healing*. New York: Routledge.
Lankauskas, G. 2006. "Sensuous (Re)Collections: The Sight and Taste of Socialism at Grutas Statue Park, Lithuania." *Senses and Society*, 1: 27–52.
Largey, G. and D. Watson. 1972. "The Sociology of Odours." *American Journal of Sociology*, 77: 1021–1034.
Law, J. and A. Mol. 1995. "Notes on Materiality and Sociality." *Sociological Review*, 43: 274–294.
Law, L. 2001. "Home Cooking: Filipino Women and the Geographies of the Senses in Hong Kong." *Cultural Geographies*, 8: 264–284.
Leder, D. 1990. *The Absent Body*. Chicago: University of Chicago Press.
LeDoux, J. 2002. *The Synaptic Self: How Our Brains Become Who We Are*. New York: Penguin Books.
Leiss, W., S. Klein, S. Jhally, and J. Botterill. 2005. *Social Communication in Advertising: Consumption in the Mediated Marketplace*. Third edition. New York: Routledge.

Leont'ev, A. 1981. *Problems of the Development of the Mind.* Moscow: Progress Publishers.

Lepecki, S. and A. Banes. 2006. "Introduction." In A. Banes and S. Lepecki (eds.), *The Senses in Performance*, 1–17. New York: Routledge.

Lévy, P. 1997. *Collective Intelligence: Mankind's Emerging World in Cyberspace.* New York: Plenum.

Lindstrom, M. 2005. *Brand Sense: Build Powerful Brands through Touch, Taste, Sight, and Sound.* New York: Simon and Schuster.

Lingis, A. 1996. *Sensation: Intelligibility in Sensibility.* New York: Humanity Books.

Lipovetsky, G. 1983. *L' Ere du Vide: Essais sur l'Individualisme Contemporain.* Paris: Gallimard.

——. 1987. "La Pub Sort Ses Griffes." *Le Débat*, 43:126–140.

——. 2005. *Hypermodern Times.* Cambridge: Polity Press.

——. 2006. *Le Bonheur Paradoxal: Essai sur la Société d'Hyperconsommation.* Paris: Gallimard.

Lorimer, H. 2005. "Cultural Geography: The Busyness of Being 'More-Than-Representational.'" *Progress in Human Geography*, 29: 83–95.

——. 2007. "Cultural Geography: Worldly Shapes, Differently Arranged." *Progress in Human Geography*, 31: 89–100.

——. 2008. "Cultural Geography: Non-Representational Conditions and Concerns." *Progress in Human Geography*, 32: 551–559.

Low, K. 2005. "Ruminations on Smell as a Sociocultural Phenomenon." *Current Sociology*, 53: 397–417.

——. 2006. "Presenting the Self, the Social Body, and the Olfactory: Managing Smells in Everyday Life Experiences." *Sociological Perspectives*, 49: 607–631.

Mags, A. and S. Guy. 2007. "Senses and the City." *Senses and Society*, 2: 133–136.

Mags, A., G. Moore, T. Cox, B. Croxford, M. Refaee, and S. Sharpies. 2007. "The 24-Hour City: Residents' Sensorial Experiences." *Senses and Society*, 2: 201–215.

Makagon, D. and M. Neumann. 2009. *Audio Documentary and the Ethnographic Experience.* Thousand Oaks, CA: SAGE.

Malnar, J. and F. Vodvarka. 2004. *Sensory Design.* Minneapolis: University of Minnesota Press.

Marks, L. 1999. *The Skin of the Film: Intercultural Cinema, Embodiment, and the Senses.* Durham, NC: Duke University Press.

Marx, K. (1967) [1844]. *The Economic and Philosophic Manuscripts of 1844.* Available online at http://www.marxists.org/archive/marx/index.htm (last accessed July 10, 2010).

Masters, W. and V. Johnson. 1966. *Human Sexual Response.* Philadelphia, PA: Lippincott Williams and Wilkins.

Maugham, S. 1930. *On a Chinese Screen.* New York: Doran.

McCarthy, D. 1984. "Toward a Sociology of the Physical World." *Studies in Symbolic Interaction*, 5: 105–121.

McKenzie, C. 2008. "Radio in/for Research: Creating Knowledge Waves." In

G. Knowles and A. Cole (eds.), *Handbook of the Arts in Qualitative Research*, 337–349. Thousand Oaks, CA: SAGE.

Mead, G.H. 1929. *The Philosophy of the Present*. Chicago: University of Chicago Press.

——. 1934. *Mind, Self, and Society*. Edited by C. Morris. Chicago: University of Chicago Press.

——. 1938. *The Philosophy of the Act*. Chicago: University of Chicago Press.

Merleau-Ponty, M. 1962. *Phenomenology of Perception*. London: Routledge.

Middleton, J. 2010. "Sense and the City: Exploring the Embodied Geographies of Urban Walking." *Social and Cultural Geography*, 11: 575–596.

Miller, D. 1987. *Material Culture and Mass Consumption*. Oxford: Blackwell.

Miller, I. 1997. *The Anatomy of Disgust*. Cambridge, MA: Harvard University Press.

Miner, H. 1956. "Body Ritual among the Nacirema." *American Anthropologist*, 58(3): 503–507.

Mitchell, R. Jr. 2002. *Dancing at Armageddon: Survivalism and Chaos in Modern Times*. Chicago: University of Chicago Press.

Morin, E. and A.B. Kern. 1993. *Terre–Patrie*. Paris: Seuil.

Mosher, D.L., M. Barton-Henry, and S. Green. 1988. "Subjective Sexual Arousal and Involvement: Development of Multiple Indicators." *Journal of Sex Research*, 25: 412–425.

Nederveen Pieterse, J. 1993. "Aesthetics of Power: Time and Body Politics." *Third Text*, 7: 33–42.

Ness, S.A.A. 2004. "Being a Body in a Cultural Way: Understanding the Cultural in the Embodiment of Dance." In H. Thomas and J. Ahmed (eds.), *Cultural Bodies: Ethnography and Theory*, 123–144. Oxford: Blackwell.

Nocke, A. 2006. "Israel and the Emergence of Mediterranean Identity: Expressions of Locality in Music and Literature." *Israel Studies*, 11: 143–173.

Norton, T. 1975. *Ordinals of Alchemy*. Oxford: Oxford University Press.

Nuckolls, J. 1999. *Sounds Like Life: Sound-Symbolic Grammar, Performance, and Cognition*. New York: Oxford University Press.

Ochs, E., C. Pontecorvo, and A. Fasulo. 1996. "Socializing Taste." *Ethnos*, 61: 7–46.

Ogletree, S.M. and H.J. Ginsburg. 2000. "Kept under the Hood: Neglect of the Clitoris in Common Vernacular." *Sex Roles*, 43: 917–926.

O'Hanlon, M. 1989. *Reading the Skin: Adornment, Display, and Society among the Wahgi*. London: British Museum.

Ong, W. 1982. *Orality and Literacy: The Technologizing of the Word*. New York: Routledge.

Oosterbaan, M. 2009. "Sonic Supremacy: Sound, Space and Charisma in a Favela in Rio de Janeiro." *Critique of Anthropology*, 29: 81–104.

Orwell, G. 1937. *The Road to Wigan Pier*. London: Victor Gollancz.

Owens, E. 2007. "Nonbiologic Objects as Actors." *Symbolic Interaction*, 30: 567–584.

Oz, Almog. 2000. *The Sabra: The Creation of the New Jew*. Berkeley: University of California Press.

Oz, Amos. 2009. *The Amos Oz Reader*. Boston, MA: Houghton Mifflin Harcourt.

Panopoulos, P. 2003. "Animal Bells as Symbols: Sound and Hearing in a Greek Island Village." *Journal of the Royal Anthropological Institute*, 9: 639–656.

Parisi, D. 2008. "'Fingerbombing,' or 'Touching is Good': The Cultural Construction of Technologized Touch." *Senses and Society*, 3: 307–327.

Paterson, M. 2009. "Haptic Geographies: Ethnography, Haptic Knowledges, and Sensuous Dispositions." *Progress in Human Geography*, 33: 766–788.

Peek, P. 1994. "The Sounds of Silence: Cross-World Communications and the Auditory Arts in African Societies." *American Ethnologist*, 21: 474–494.

Peirce, C.S. 1931. *Collected Writings*. Volumes 1–8. Cambridge, MA: Harvard University Press.

Pelias, R. 1999. *Writing Performance: Poeticizing the Researcher's Body*. Carbondale: Southern Illinois University Press.

Penslar, D. 2003. "Transmitting Jewish Culture: Radio in Israel." *Jewish Social Studies*, 10: 1–29.

Peynaud, E. 2005. "Tasting Problems and Errors of Perception." In C. Korsmeyer (ed.), *The Taste Culture Reader*, 272–278. Oxford: Berg.

Piesse, C.H. 1891. *Piesse's Art of Perfumery*. London: Piesse & Ludin.

Pilowsky, A.L. 1985. "Yiddish alongside the Revival of Hebrew: Public Polemics on the Status of Yiddish in Eretz Israel 1907–1921." In J. Fishman (ed.), *Readings in the Sociology of Jewish Languages*, 104–124. Amsterdam: E.J. Brill.

Pink, S. 2006. *The Future of Visual Anthropology: Engaging the Senses*. London: Routledge.

——. 2008. "An Urban Tour: The Sensory Sociality of Ethnographic Place-Making." *Ethnography*, 9: 175–196.

Plante, R. 2006. *Sexualities in Context: A Social Perspective*. Boulder, CO: Westview.

Porteous, D. 2006. "Smellscape." In J. Drobnick (ed.), *The Smell Culture Reader*, 89–106. Oxford: Berg.

Potter, C. 2008. "Senses of Motion, Senses of Self: Becoming a Dancer." *Ethnos*, 73: 444–465.

Presner, T. 2003. "'Clear Heads, Solid Stomachs, and Hard Muscles': Max Nordau and the Aesthetics of Jewish Regeneration." *Modernism/Modernity*, 10: 269–296.

——. 2006. "Muscle Jews and Airplanes: Modernist Mythologies, the Great War, and the Politics of Regeneration." *Modernism/Modernity*, 13: 701–728.

Proust, M. 2001 [1913–1927]. *In Search of Lost Time*. New York: Random House.

Rapoport, T., E. Lomsky-Feder, and A. Heider. 2002. "Recollection and Relocation in Immigration: Russian-Jewish Immigrants Normalize Their Anti-Semitic Experiences." *Symbolic Interaction*, 25: 175–198.

Regan, P. 1997. "The Impact of Male Sexual Request Style on Perceptions of Sexual Interactions: The Mediational Role of Beliefs about Female Sexual Desire." *Basic and Applied Social Psychology*, 19: 519–532.

Regan, P. and E. Berscheid. 1999. *Lust: What We Know about Human Sexual Desire*. Thousand Oaks, CA: SAGE.

Regev, M. 1996. "Musica Mizrakhit, Israeli Rock and National Culture in Israel Popular Music." *Middle East Issues*, 15: 275–284.

Rheingold, H. 1992. *Virtual Reality*. New York: Touchstone.
Rice, T. 2003. "Soundselves: An Acoustemology of Sound and Self in the Edinburgh Royal Infirmary." *Anthropology Today*, 19: 4–10.
Ritchel, M. 2010a. "Digital Devices Deprive Brain of Needed Downtime." *New York Times*, August 24.
——. 2010b. "Hooked on Gadgets and Paying a Mental Price." *New York Times*, June 6.
Robbins, K. 1994. "Forces of Consumption: From the Symbolic to the Psychotic." *Media Culture and Society*, 16: 449–468.
Rochberg-Halton, E. 1982. "Qualitative Immediacy and the Communicative Act." *Qualitative Sociology*, 5: 162–181.
Rodaway, P. 1994. *Sensuous Geographies: Body, Sense, and Place*. London: Routledge.
Roseman, M. 1993. *Healing Sounds from the Malaysian Rainforest: Temiar Music and Medicine*. Thousand Oaks: University of California Press.
Rozin, P., J. Haidt, and C. McCauley. 1993. "Digust." In M. Lewis and J. Havilland (eds.), *Handbook of Emotions*, 575–594. New York: Guilford Press.
Rye, B.J. and G. Meaney. 2007. "The Pursuit of Sexual Pleasure." *Sexuality and Culture*, 11: 28–51.
Schab, F. and R. Crowder (eds.). 1995. *Memory for Odors*. Mahwah, NJ: Lawrence Erlbaum.
Schechner, R. 2002. *Performance Studies: An Introduction*. New York: Routledge.
——. 2003. *Performance Theory*. New York: Routledge.
——. 2006. "Rasaesthetics." In S. Banes and A. Lepecki (eds.), *The Senses in Performance*, 19–34. New York: Routledge.
Schieffelin, E. 1985. "Performance and the Cultural Construction of Reality." *American Ethnologist*, 12: 707–724.
Schwartz, B. 1991. "Social Change and Collective Memory: The Democratization of George Washington." *American Sociological Review*, 56: 221–236.
Schwartz, B., Y. Zerubavel, and B. Barnett. 1996. "The Recovery of Masada: A Study in Collective Memory." *Sociological Quarterly*, 27: 147–164.
Searle, J. 1968. *Speech Acts: A Study in the Philosophy of Language*. Cambridge: Cambridge University Press.
Seeger, A. 1975. "The Meaning of Body Ornaments: A Suya Example." *Ethnology*, 14: 211–224.
——. 1979. "What Can We Learn When They Sing? Vocal Genres of the Suya Indians of Central Brazil." *Ethnomusicology*, 23: 373–394.
Serematakis, N. (ed.). 1994. *The Senses Still: Perception as Memory and Material Culture in Modernity*. Boulder, CO: Westview.
Serres, M. 2008. *Five Senses*. New York: Continuum.
Sheller, M. 2004. "Automotive Emotions: Feeling the Car." *Theory Culture and Society*, 21: 221–242.
Shepard, P. 1992. *Nature and Madness*. San Francisco, CA: Sierra Club Books.
Shilling, C. 1993. *The Body and Social Theory*. London: SAGE.
Simmel, G. 1950. *The Sociology of Georg Simmel*. Edited by K. Wolff. New York: Free Press.

——. 1997. *Simmel on Culture*. Edited by David Frisby and Mike Featherstone. Thousand Oaks, CA: SAGE.

Smith, M. 2007. *Sensory History: An Introduction*. Oxford: Berg.

Snow, D. and L. Anderson. 1987. "Identity Work among the Homeless." *American Journal of Sociology*, 92: 1336–1371.

Sparkes, A.C. 2009. "Ethnography and the Senses: Challenges and Possibilities." *Qualitative Research in Sport and Exercise*, 1: 21–35.

Spenser, E. 1989. *The Yale Edition of the Shorter Poems of Edmund Spenser*. New Haven, CT: Yale University Press.

Sprinzak, E. 1987. "From Messianic Pioneering to Vigilante Terrorism: The Case of the Gush Emunim Underground." *Journal of Strategic Studies*, 10: 194–216.

Sterne, J. 2001. "Mediate Auscultation, the Stethoscope, and the Autopsy of the Living: Medicine's Acoustic Culture." *Journal of Medical Humanities*, 22: 115–136.

Stoddart, D.M. 1990. *The Scented Ape*. Cambridge: Cambridge University Press.

Stokes, R. and P. Hewitt. 1976. "Aligning Actions." *American Sociological Review*, 41: 838–849.

Stoller, P. 1984. "Sound in Songhay Cultural Experience." *American Ethnologist*, 11: 559–570.

——. 1989. *Taste of Ethnographic Things: The Senses in Anthropology*. Philadelphia: University of Pennsylvania Press.

——. 1997. *Sensuous Scholarship*. Philadelphia: University of Pennsylvania Press.

——. 2004. "Sensuous Ethnography, African Persuasion, and Social Knowledge." *Qualitative Inquiry*, 10: 817–835.

Stone, G. 1962. "Appearance and the Self." In A. Rose (ed.), *Human Behavior and Social Processes*, 86–118. Boston, MA: Houghton Mifflin.

Stroeken, K. 2008. "Sensory Shifts and Synaesthetics in Sukuma Healing." *Ethnos*, 73: 466–484.

Suler, J. 1996. "Psychology of Cyberspace." Available online at http://www.enotalone.com/article/2454.html (last accessed December 30, 2010).

Sullivan, L. 1986. "Sound and Senses: Toward a Hermeneutic of Performance." *History of Religions*, 26: 1–33.

——. 2008. "Painting as Research: Create and Critique." In G. Knowles and A. Cole (eds.), *Handbook of the Arts in Qualitative Research: Perspectives, Methodologies, Examples, and Issues*, 239–250. Thousand Oaks, CA: SAGE.

Summers, M. 1956. *The History of Witchcraft and Demonology*. New York: University Books.

Sutton, D. 2001. *Remembrance of Repasts: An Anthropology of Food and Memory*. Oxford: Berg.

Synnott, A. 1991. "A Sociology of Smell." *Canadian Review of Sociology and Anthropology*, 28: 437–459.

——. 1993. *The Body Social: Symbolism, Self, and Society*. London: Routledge.

Tarr, R. 1996. *South West Coast Path: Minehead to Padstow*. London: Aurum Press.

Thompson, C. 1969 [1927]. *The Mystery and Lure of Perfume*. Detroit, MI: Singing Tree.

Thrift, N. 2003. "Performance and . . ." *Environment and Planning A*, 35: 2019–2024.
——. 2008. *Non-Representational Theory: Space, Politics, Affect*. London: Routledge.
Thrift, N. and J.D. Dewsbury. 2000. "Dead Geographies and How to Make Them Live." *Environment and Planning D*, 18: 411–432.
Tilley, C. 2006a. "Objectification." In C. Tilley, W. Keane, S. Kuechler-Fogden, M. Rowlands, and P. Spyer (eds.), *Handbook of Material Culture*, 60–73. London: SAGE.
——. 2006b. "The Sensory Dimensions of Gardening." *Senses and Society*, 3: 311–330.
Tolman, D. 1994. "Doing Desire: Adolescent Girls' Struggles for/with Sexuality." *Gender and Society*, 8(3): 324–342.
Tuan, Y.F. 2001. *Space and Place: The Perspective of Experience*. Minneapolis: University of Minnesota Press.
Turner, V. 1969. *The Ritual Process: Structure and Anti-Structure*. Ithaca, NY: Cornell University Press.
——. 1974. *Dramas, Fields, and Metaphors: Symbolic Action in Human Society*. Ithaca, NY: Cornell University Press.
Turner, V. and R. Schechner. 1988. *The Anthropology of Performance*. New York: PAJ.
Tyler, S. 1986. "Postmodern Ethnography: From Document of the Occult, to Occult Document." In J. Cliford and G. Marcus (eds.), *Writing Culture: The Poetics and Politics of Ethnography*, 122–140. Berkeley: University of California Press.
Urry, J. 2000. *Sociology beyond Societies*. New York: Routledge.
——. 2007. *Mobilities*. Cambridge: Polity Press.
van Gennep, A. 1909. *The Rites of Passage*. London: Routledge and Kegan Paul.
Van Leeuwen, T. 1999. *Speech, Music, Sound*. London: Palgrave Macmillan.
Van Maanen, J. 1988. *Tales of the Field: On Writing Ethnography*. Chicago: University of Chicago Press.
Vannini, P. and A. McCright. 2004. "To Die for: The Semiotic Seductive Power of the Tanned Body." *Symbolic Interaction*, 27: 309–332.
Vannini, P. and D. Waskul. 2006. "Body Image beyond Dualism." In D. Waskul and P. Vannini (eds.), *Body/Embodiment: Symbolic Interaction and the Sociology of the Body*, 183–200. Aldershot: Ashgate.
Vannini, P., D. Waskul, S. Gottschalk, and T. Ellis. Forthcoming. "Making Sense of the Weather: Dwelling and Weathering on Canada's Rain Coast." *Space and Culture*.
Volosinov, V. 1973. *Marxism and the Philosophy of Language*. New York: Seminar Press.
Warren, S. 2008. "Empirical Challenges in Organizational Aesthetics Research: Towards a Sensual Methodology." *Organization Studies*, 29: 559–580.
Waskul, D. 2003. *Self-Games and Body-Play: Personhood in Online Chat and Cybersex*. New York: Peter Lang.
——. 2009. "'My Boyfriend Loves it When I Come Home from This Class': Pedagogy, Titillation, and New Media Technologies." *Sexualities*, 12: 654–661.
Waskul, D. and P. Van der Riet. 2002. "The Abject Embodiment of Cancer Patients: Dignity, Selfhood, and the Grotesque Body." *Symbolic Interaction*, 25: 487–513.

Waskul, D. and P. Vannini. 2008. "Smell, Odor, and Somatic Work: Sense-Making and Sensory Management." *Social Psychology Quarterly*, 71: 53–71.
Waskul, D. and M. Waskul. 2009. "Paddle and Portage: The *Travail* of BWCA Canoe Travel." In P. Vannini (ed.), *The Cultures of Alternative Mobility*, 21–37. Aldershot: Ashgate.
Waskul, D., P. Vannini, and D. Wiesen. 2007. "Women and Their Clitoris: Personal Discovery, Signification, and Use." *Symbolic Interaction*, 30: 151–174.
Waskul, D., P. Vannini, and J. Wilson. 2009. "The Aroma of Recollection: Olfaction, Nostalgia, and the Shaping of the Sensuous Self." *Senses and Society*, 4: 5–22.
Weigert, A.J. 1997. *Self, Interaction, and Natural Environment: Refocusing our Eyesight.* Albany: State University of New York Press.
Weinberg, M. and C. Williams. 2005. "Fecal Matters: Habitus, Embodiments, and Deviance." *Social Problems*, 52: 315–336.
Weinstein, D. 2000. *Heavy Metal.* New York: Da Capo Press.
Weinstein, E. and P. Deutschberger. 1963. "Some Dimensions of Altercasting." *Sociometry*, 26: 454–466.
Weissbrod, L. 1982. "Gush Emunim Ideology: From Religious Doctrine to Political Action." *Middle Eastern Studies*, 18: 265–275.
——. 1996. "Gush Emunim and the Peace Process: Modern Religious Fundamentalism in Crisis." *Israel Affairs*, 3: 86–103.
Welters, L. 1995. "Ethnicity in Greek Dress." In J. Eicher (ed.), *Ethnicity and Dress*, 53–77. Oxford: Berg.
Wernick, A. 1997. "Resort to Nostalgia: Mountains, Memories, and Myths of Time." In M. Nava, A. Blake, I. MacRury, and B. Richards (eds.), *Buy This Book: Studies in Advertising and Consumption*, 207–223. New York: Routledge.
Wiggins, S. 2002. "Talking with Your Mouth Full: Gustatory Mmms and the Embodiment of Pleasure." *Research on Language and Social Interaction*, 35: 311–336.
Williams, G. and S. Bendelow. 1998. *The Lived Body: Sociological Themes, Embodied Issues.* London: Routledge.
Willis, P. 1978. *Profane Culture.* London: Routledge.
Wright. L. 2003. *Clean and Decent: The Fascinating History of the Bathroom and Water Closet.* New York: Penguin.
Wylie, J. 2002. "An Essay on Ascending Glastonbury Tor." *Geoforum*, 33: 441–454.
——. 2005. "A Single Day's Walking: Narrating Self and Landscape on the South West Coast Path." *Transactions of the Institute of British Geographers*, 30(NS): 234–247.
Zamponi, S. 1997. *Fascist Spectacle: The Aesthetics of Power in Mussolini's Italy.* Berkeley: University of California Press.
Zerubavel, E. 1991. *The Fine Line: Making Distinctions in Everyday Life.* Chicago: University of Chicago Press.
——. 1996. "Lumping and Splitting: Notes on Social Classification." *Sociological Forum*, 11: 421–433.

INDEX

For Product Safety Concerns and Information please contact our EU
representative GPSR@taylorandfrancis.com
Taylor & Francis Verlag GmbH, Kaufingerstraße 24, 80331 München, Germany

www.ingramcontent.com/pod-product-compliance
Ingram Content Group UK Ltd.
Pitfield, Milton Keynes, MK11 3LW, UK
UKHW022354190926
475702UK00015B/2281

* 9 7 8 0 4 1 5 7 3 1 0 4 1 *